Is Your HEALTH CARE KILLING YOU?

Is Your HEALTH CARE KILLING YOU?

12 Ways to Survive Our Fractured Health Care System

Colleen C. Badell, Ph.D.

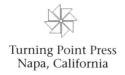

Turning Point Press
Napa, California

Turning Point Press
P.O. Box 4111
Napa, California 94558–0411

Copyright © 2006 by Colleen C. Badell, Ph.D.

All rights reserved.
Published 2006 by Turning Point Press.

No part of this book may be reproduced or transmitted in any form or by any means, electronic or mechanical, including photocopying, recording, or by any information storage and retrieval system, without permission in writing from the publisher.

Printed in the United States of America

For more information, visit www.health-advocate.com

Interior typesetting by Desktop Miracles, Inc.
Index by Linzer Indexing Services
Cartoons rendered by Erin Leong

Library of Congress Control Number 2004098526
ISBN 0–9761129–2–2

CIP data available

The author has made every effort to ensure the accuracy of information contained in the book and to give proper credit where warranted. Any omissions or errors are unintentional.

Examples contained in this book are versions of actual consumer occurrences derived from clinical case files and first-hand accounts of events and circumstances. Names, locations, and other identifying data have been intentionally omitted to preserve the anonymity and protect the privacy of those involved.

Contents

CHAPTER 1	The Health Care Battleground	9
CHAPTER 2	Assume An Active Role	25
CHAPTER 3	Are You a Health Care Victim?	37
CHAPTER 4	Be Selective About Providers	45
CHAPTER 5	Prepare for Appointments	63
CHAPTER 6	Assert Yourself with Providers	71
CHAPTER 7	Do Your Own Research	83
CHAPTER 8	Engage in Health Self-Care	93
CHAPTER 9	Connect with Medical Support Staff	101
CHAPTER 10	Network with Other Consumers	109
CHAPTER 11	Request Copies of Records & Reports	113
CHAPTER 12	Track Your Own Progress	119
CHAPTER 13	Exercise Patience with Results	123
CHAPTER 14	Know Your Health Care Rights	129
CHAPTER 15	Prepare for Emergencies	145
CHAPTER 16	Conclusion	155

IS YOUR HEALTH CARE KILLING YOU?

APPENDIX A	State Agencies & Licensing Boards	167
APPENDIX B	Consumer Advocacy Groups, Health Rights Organizations, & Medical Information Services	181
APPENDIX C	Professional Associations & Organizations	183

Bibliography   189

Index   195

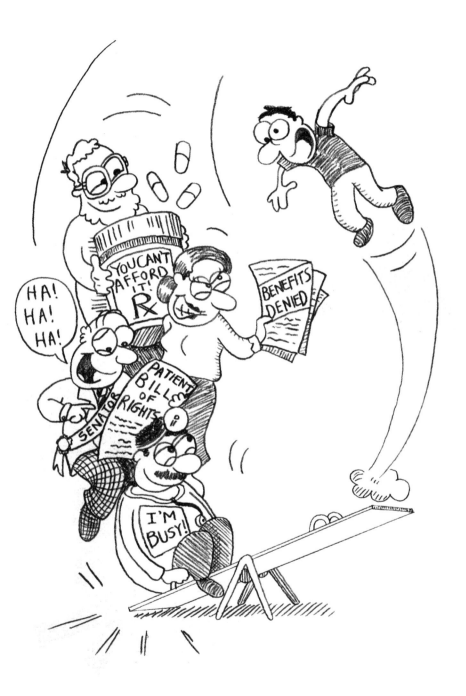

*It's a funny thing about life;
If you refuse to accept anything but the best,
you very often get it.*

W. SOMERSET MAUGHAM

1

The Health Care Battleground

In a complicated health care environment of insurance company limitations, preventable medical mistakes, and high demand for more natural treatments, not to mention constant environmental threats to health and safety and an extended life expectancy, it is essential that we take more and more responsibility for our own health.

The conventional medicine industry has become consumed with profit and a gatekeeper mentality, which seeks to dictate to consumers what we should and should not receive in health care. Financial incentives and high costs complicate the priorities of the industry, creating a highly competitive environment for your consumer dollar. This environment demands the evolution of an involved health care consumer.

It is no wonder that regulators and providers are locked in a tug of war over control for your care. Regulators make money when people *do not* get treatment, and providers make money when people *do* get treatment. Insurance companies complain about unnecessary treatment and rising medical costs. Providers complain about loss of control and reduced payment for services. Care you need is denied by regulators. The quality of care received from providers has gotten worse. This battle brings legislators into the fray.

Health care is often described as the "world's largest service industry." Somewhere along the way, the quality of service offered to people has irreparably suffered as the focus has shifted from serving consumers to using consumers. This change has been so gradual that we barely notice it, giving the health care industry relative impunity for their exploitive actions and creating a precarious environment for the person whose health is already at stake. Unfortunately, this focus has made our system of medicine as threatening to people as the illness it treats. In the process of serving the interests of regulators, providers, and legislators, the interests of the consumer get lost.

Just how bad the health industry has become is exemplified in one consumer's experience. Every year, this consumer contacts her insurer to find out exactly what services are included in the annual physical examination. She does this to avoid confusion because, every year, her insurer pays fewer and fewer benefits, which are documented in complicated addendums to her family's policy.

One year, the insurer denied payment for four out of five preventive services because of the following: misinformation about a benefit, two claims processing errors, incorrect coding submitted on two tests, and the wrong test ordered by the provider, all of which resulted in unjustified charges to the consumer totaling $170. Two of the errors occurred on a single test whose contracted rate was a measly $4.49. It took two months to resolve all the mistakes and over one month to secure the radiology reports, which were sent to two wrong doctors after three requests and repeated contact with three hospital departments.

To put all this in perspective, this consumer pays premiums of over $16,000 annually for herself and her spouse and out-of-pocket costs in the range of $10,000–$20,000 annually for preventive alternative medicine services. This couple only use their health plan for annual physical exams. All of the problems outlined above arose from a single preventive visit to the doctor for what was supposed to be no more than a $30 co-payment. Imagine what the experience would be if a person was really sick!

The fact that health care continues to fail to meet the needs of consumers is abundantly clear. The big business of medicine, high price of technology, price-gouging of pharmaceutical companies, medical malpractice lawsuits, insurance company interference, provider arrogance and greed, medical specialization, and consumer complacency have all been alternately or simultaneously blamed for our current health care crisis. These circumstances exist for good reason.

First, it is what happens when you apply capitalism to health care and it is allowed to run amok. An out-of-control capitalism blinds us into thinking that just because we *can* do something, we *should* do it, particularly if there is money to be made and regardless of the cost to others. We did not invent materialism, but we have certainly elevated it to new heights by condoning it under morally questionable circumstances, making it socially acceptable to flaunt it, and pitying those who fail to share our view. A cash register mentality creates a myopic approach to health care and a decided preference for what you can get away with or what is legal over what is right.

The ironies are obvious. We create the very adversarial environment that we then champion people to overcome. We base our entire system of health care on profit and then wonder why it has become so corrupt.

Capitalism both institutionalizes and commercializes medicine, turning our health care system into an infinite sea of corporations. Institutionalized medicine results in assembly line treatment in which individual needs are overlooked or ignored—the single worst development in modern medical history—and a massive, outdated bureaucracy that impedes the healing process.

Ralph Nader accused corporate America of "commercializing everything it touches." Corporate health care is no exception to this rule. Along with the problems associated with institutionalized medicine, we must also now contend with medical elitism, in which only the rich receive the best care.

Alternative medicine is falling prey to this environment as it gains more and more acceptance and is incorporated into our conventional system of medicine. It is also becoming increasingly subject to regulation, which will result in its application to a mass audience without adequate consideration for individual needs. Many alternative practices are beginning to organize into associations to set standards for practice, disseminate information, and make referrals to the public, and some practices are licensed by state governments. Nutritional supplements are now termed nutraceuticals, echoing the pharmaceuticals of conventional medicine, and may soon find themselves targeted for more comprehensive government regulation.

Either alternative providers refuse to accept insurance payments or their services are not eligible for reimbursement. Also, those who are popular typically charge exorbitant fees. Few discounts are offered for cash payment or economic hardship, causing people to pay high costs for alternative treatments and therapies.

Personal wealth means better conventional care, and personal wealth now means better alternative care. Alternative medicine is beginning to sound and act just like conventional medicine. This is a sure sign that we are heading toward a generic system of medical practice in which only the type of medicine that is applied will differ.

There are not just economic inequities in health care but gender and racial ones as well. For decades, there has been a gross lack of research funding for women's health issues. Hormonal replacement therapy (HRT), whose usage dates from World War II, was only recently the object of a large-scale study to examine its long-term consequences. Attention-Deficit/Hyperactivity Disorder (ADHD) in women is only now being examined.

A recent report by the Institute of Medicine found that blacks, Hispanics, and other minorities received lower quality health care than whites, and a study on Medicare-managed plans found that white people get better treatment than blacks for mental illness and other disorders. Surveys point to the fact that there are few alternative medicine providers or services in ethnic neighborhoods.

Is Your Health Care Killing You?

The business of medicine has become a huge industry. National health expenditures rose to $1.55 trillion in 2002, three times the national defense budget and almost 15% of the gross domestic product (GDP). By 2013, this figure is expected to more than double to $3.4 trillion, outpacing economic growth and creating a huge burden on consumers. An increasingly older population with age-related health issues will add to this burden, as will an over-reliance on high-priced medical technology, leading to its misuse.

Our dependence on all forms of technology for more than one hundred years is also taking its toll on our health as environmentally induced illness becomes more and more prevalent. Once thought to be only for our benefit, technology, as it turns out, has many harmful consequences.

The pharmaceutical industry is the richest industry in America today. One estimate is that it is more than five times more profitable than the average for Fortune 500 companies. Pharmaceutical companies have been accused of price-gouging customers, reporting only positive outcomes from research and concealing negative ones, delaying the introduction of generic versions of brand name drugs, representing drugs as new when they are only duplications of cheaper ones already on the market, and engaging in other misleading marketing tactics.

Pharmaceutical companies charge high prices for the same prescription drugs that cost a fraction of the price in places such as Canada, Europe, and Mexico. Why? Federal patent protection guarantees pharmaceutical company profits by eliminating competition for an extended period of time.

Many people, especially senior citizens on a budget, have resorted to purchasing prescription drugs in other countries, where patent protections run out much earlier and drugs are 50%–85% less costly. For example, Lamisil®, a brand name drug for fungal infections, costs $300 for a 30-day supply in the U.S., but the generic version, made in Canada and sold in Brazil, costs only $55 for the same 30-day supply. There are now many online pharmacies that are based in other countries but fill U.S. prescriptions via the Internet and by regular mail.

Pharmaceutical companies claim that they need to charge high prices to pay for research and development, but industry sources counter that drug companies spend more money on marketing and sales than on research and development. In fact, critics claim that there is a distinct correlation between rising drugs costs and direct-to-consumer advertising and that the National Institutes of Health (NIH) pays for more than one-third of all medical research.

What pharmaceutical companies fail to acknowledge is that they spend millions of dollars on lobbying efforts to keep them free from federal regulation, which would force them to lower the costs of prescription drugs. In 2003, they spent almost five million dollars to lobby the Food and Drug Administration alone, creating a conflict of interest that many critics characterize as "the fox in charge of the henhouse." Drug companies also use loopholes in federal patent protection law in order to delay the introduction of less-expensive generic drugs into the marketplace.

Nutritional supplements and herbal medicines are less regulated than prescription drugs, so alternative medicine manufacturers are free to make huge profits with considerable variations in the quality of products.

The insurance industry has a veritable choke-hold on health care, fostering a state of perpetual competition between insurers and providers, particularly in managed care. The traditional fee for service basis of private health plans encourages providers to order unnecessary tests and procedures because they are paid for the number of services ordered. At the same time, the fixed rates imposed by HMO capitated care discourage necessary tests and procedures because providers are paid a flat rate regardless of the number of services ordered. The choice is incentive to provide unnecessary care versus incentive to provide less care. In both instances, the consumer loses. Third-party involvement results either in deficient care or harm if consumers are denied the care they need.

We are paying more than we ever have before for health insurance but are getting fewer and fewer benefits. Premiums for health plans jumped 13.9% in 2003, the third year of double-digit growth and the biggest spike since 1990. Where does all the money go that you and your employer pay to insurance companies for health benefits? Industry critics claim that the majority of your insurance premium is allocated toward administration and stockholder profits rather than the actual payment of benefits.

Not only is your care compromised by regulators but so is your medical privacy. Third-party access to and inappropriate use of confidential medical records compromise the privacy that should rightfully exist between providers and their patients. Many people feel they can no longer afford to be totally honest with their provider if the information will be used against them by their insurer to deny benefits or to increase premiums. Medical information technologies such as Internet access to confidential medical records may threaten your medical privacy even further.

There can be no question that insurance companies with their profit priority have lowered the quality of health care in our country. Managed care was created to serve the financial bottom line, not to improve the quality of care.

Many experts cite the millions of people who have no health insurance whatsoever as the major problem in health care (an increasing one according to a recent Census Bureau report, making uninsurance not just a problem of the poor). The real problem, however, lies with the insurers themselves. The fact that serious medical decisions are made by regulators with no medical training whatsoever makes their very existence questionable and should be the primary object of health care reform. On the other hand, should health decisions be placed solely in the hands of providers who only profit when people are ill?

The healers of the past were never wealthy nor were they ever intended to be, and it is a ghoulish notion that doctors profit from the pain and suffering of their patients and care more about maintaining a lifestyle than helping you to get well. Either scenario constitutes a dual relationship, which encourages an emphasis on quantity over quality and compromises our care. It is a conflict of interest that is almost never discussed in any serious conversation about health care reform, and we tacitly accept it as a normal part of life without ever questioning its impact on us.

There are no limitations on what health care providers charge for their services, but most people would agree that they charge too much. According to the American Medical Association, medical doctors earn about six times the salary of the average worker. Despite this fact, it is the rare doctor who offers a sliding fee scale to the economically disadvantaged or a reasonable cash discount to customers who want to pay up front for medical services. More and more providers refuse to accept patients on low-income, government-supported health programs or accept insurance payments due to the headaches associated with managed care. Nowhere is provider greed more evident than in Medicare fraud, which is estimated to cost taxpayers $20 billion per year.

It has been established in studies that medical doctors overprescribe tests and procedures in which they have a financial interest. It would then follow that providers who sell products for a profit are also more inclined to recommend those products to consumers. Once only the province of plastic surgeons, health providers today hawk everything from skin care products to eye surgery to herbs and supplements.

Questions have recently been raised about oncologists, or cancer specialists, the majority of whose revenue is derived from substantial markups on chemotherapy drugs that are administered in the office. This obvious conflict of interest has been loudly criticized within the medical profession.

Medical elitism has recently reached new heights in the form of VIP medical care, also termed "boutique medicine." Beginning in the 1990s, two elite medical services established themselves in health care: MDVIP based in Florida and MD2 based in Washington, both with franchises in several states. VIP medical services charge clients anywhere from $1,500 to $20,000 per year above the normal costs of health insurance policies for preferential treatment such as doctors' personal cell phone numbers, home delivery of medicines, and same day appointments with no wait or rush.

Many providers have simply discarded the traditional system and replaced it with *less access* by eliminating HMO benefits and using nurse practitioners and other support staff to take histories, make referrals, and renew prescriptions. Others have replaced it with *more access* in the form of house calls, email communications, same day service, and 24-hour on-call service.

Many of these reinstated services of old come with new high premiums. One medical practice charges $350 annually for email access. One provider claimed that he would accept 50% of his fees if paid at the time of service. Since eliminating insurance benefits, he now charges patients $50 for only ten minutes of his time, suggesting that he previously billed insurance companies $600 per hour?

Any financial incentive attached to health care compromises the quality of care that consumers receive. In a managed care climate, providers do have to contend with a variety of frustrating circumstances, including complicated billing procedures and severely reduced rates for service, but they also unrealistically want to engage in a dual role of making money and helping people to get well without having to answer to anyone for their actions.

A good example of this is the hot-button issue of medical malpractice claims, which have reportedly increased the cost of insurance for doctors and hospitals to billions of dollars annually. Medical doctors regularly complain about malpractice awards, alleging that they result in higher health care costs and demanding that the federal government set award limits. But health care costs are not lower in states that have set award limits.

The position of medical doctors on this issue is also reactive rather than proactive because few doctors are willing to take the necessary steps to clean up their profession in order to reduce the likelihood of errors in the first place. The sad truth is that doctors are notorious for protecting their own, even the bad ones, and substandard doctors are rarely disciplined by licensing boards and medical societies unless their mistakes are fatal.

The government's willingness to appease doctors by limiting malpractice awards actually penalizes consumers before they are ever heard. This pre-emptive action ignores the need to identify and properly discipline offending providers *before* they cause serious harm. Also, medical malpractice claims valued at less than six figures typically never make it to court because legal costs preclude most competent attorneys from taking them, and insurers frequently fight even legitimate claims to the bitter end, making litigation too costly for the average consumer to pursue and causing more claims to fall by the wayside.

There are certainly many legitimate cases of medical negligence and incompetence, but there are also consumers, encouraged by unscrupulous personal injury attorneys, who are unable to discern true medical negligence from simply a bad medical outcome, for which no one is to blame. This "us versus them" atmosphere serves no one and does little to engender trust in the health care relationship, particularly when doctors demand liability waivers in advance of treatment.

Surveys suggest that an alarmingly high number of medical mistakes are committed every year that result in death or injury, beneficial health services are neglected, and the performance of unnecessary procedures is commonplace, particularly in the last stages of life. Study after study shows that medical treatment is disorganized, inconsistent, and fails to meet professional standards. Not only are consumers threatened by the prospect of physical injury from medical error, but they also risk harm from the negative atmosphere created by busy medical offices, clinics, and hospitals. Should we be surprised that the majority of the population use alternative medicine against the advice of the conventional medical establishment?

As we know, the medical profession likes to perpetuate the image of the prosperous, sage-like doctor who is always in control. This doctor-always-knows-best attitude has come at the expense of the needs of consumers in more areas than medical mistakes. Medical decisions frequently omit consideration for all outcomes of treatment as well as a person's ability to effect change in his own condition.

Medical specialization is one of the reasons for this tunnel vision aspect of medicine. Approximately two-thirds of all doctors in America are medical specialists. They dominate health care and earn considerably higher incomes than general practitioners or family doctors. This trend toward medical specialization has caused a critical shortage of general practitioners in our country, a trend which is expected to continue.

Medical specialization may be good for doctors, but it can be bad for consumers. One woman had severe, chronic pains in her hip and shoulder after an injury to her spine. Eleven specialists—six chiropractors and five osteopaths—misdiagnosed the condition, treating everything from muscle sprain to foot problems to no avail. Finally, a new osteopath discovered that a dislocated rib was the source of the problem, which could have been corrected in only a few visits but which was now problematic due to the passage of so much time. Treatment had spanned six years at a total out-of-pocket cost to the patient of $30,000.

Unfortunately, this is not an unusual experience for health care consumers. Health care providers, particularly specialists, seem to have trouble focusing on more than one body part at a time. When they fail to solve the problem, there are no refunds for nonperformance because providers are unfairly exempt from the same checks and balances as other profit-based businesses.

No one doubts that health care providers are overwhelmed by having to keep abreast of the latest medical developments, stay current with increasing consumer demands for more natural, less invasive treatments, and survive the cost-cutting measures of managed care and high costs of malpractice insurance. But should these be acceptable excuses for substandard care? This competitive environment also discourages providers from making appropriate referrals and collaborating with one another to provide consumers with more comprehensive care.

Getting the conventional and alternative medicine communities to work together to provide more comprehensive care is a little like trying to mix oil with water. Conventional medicine still fiercely competes with its new rival for the consumer dollar, and the majority of conventional providers simply do not support the use of alternative medicine. Since little is still known about how alternative medicine actually works, consumers are forced to find effective treatments through frustrating trial and error without much encouragement, support, or information from the conventional medical establishment.

The politicization of health care has enormous consequences for the consumer. Regulators believe that providers are the problem, wanting more services for their patients than are really necessary. Providers believe that regulators are the problem, denying services that their patients need. Other powerful interest groups like pharmaceutical companies want to maintain the status quo.

They all turn to legislators to justify and protect their selfish positions.

This battleground gives politicians and strong insurance, physician, and pharmaceutical lobbies great power over our lives as they dictate to us what to do. To a certain extent, their very existence is dependent on convincing us that they know more about our health than we do. It also results in a type of medical tyranny over the consumer and has made the entire health care process much more complicated than it should be.

The truth is that legislators, regulators, providers, and pharmaceutical companies are all part of the problem. Government involvement in personal health choices, regulators denying needed care, physicians providing substandard or inadequate care, and price-gouging pharmaceutical companies are all having an adverse effect on our health. We are also part of the problem because we allow them to get away with it. We must become more active consumers in order to be heard above these powerful voices.

Radical action seems warranted when you consider that:

- Americans receive only half the proper care they need regardless of their insurance coverage;
- 18,000 people die every year because they lack access to adequate care;
- of the 243 million people who are insured, many are denied necessary treatment due to the limitations of managed care;
- 45 million Americans (one out of every seven persons) have no health insurance whatsoever, and 11 million children are uninsured;

- 65 million Americans are without prescription drug coverage;
- alternative medicine, which is unregulated, expensive, and confusing to the consumer, has the potential for harm if not used properly.

By the year 2150, the United Nations Population Division estimates that one-third of the world's population will be over 60 years old, totaling two billion seniors and outnumbering the world's youths. They surmise that these cataclysmic numbers will cause a global economic crisis. National budgets will be stretched to the limit, straining to provide health care and other benefits to the elderly. In the absence of dramatic political reform in health policy, the grim prediction of most experts is that health care will get much worse before it gets better in our country.

Congress continues to debate the passage of a comprehensive patient Bill of Rights, which excludes the right to health care. Even if some modified version of the bill eventually becomes law, it will be the equivalent of a tiny Band-Aid on a gaping wound. The system is not flawed; it is fractured. The only chance for getting decent care lies with you, the consumer. Only by becoming educated and alert and taking as active a role as you can will you possibly get the care you deserve.

2

Assume An Active Role

The only way to take charge of your health is to assume an active role in the health care process. This requires a certain amount of effort on your part. There are twelve steps you can take to assume this role, which have arisen out of my thirty years on the frontlines of consumer advocacy in health care. These steps will give you the tools you need, but it is up to you to know what to do with them and how to apply them safely, effectively, and responsibly. Becoming a better health care consumer involves changing your approach to health care. This is *health care with an attitude!*

It is estimated that only 25–35% of the population is actually health conscious. This low figure may reflect people's mistaken belief that health is not a concern until it is lost and that health care costs are paid by employers and insurance companies. Even if employers pay premiums and insurers pay benefits, you still pay health costs in the form of deductibles and copayments. With alternative medicine you usually assume the full costs yourself.

Health consciousness used to be only the domain of the chronically and critically ill. Now that employers are cutting back on health insurance, hospital costs are escalating, the use of alternative therapies is increasing, and health information is readily available on the Internet and in other media, health consciousness is bound to grow.

Failing to assume an active role in your care may be hazardous to your health. A well-known report from the National Academy of Sciences, released in 1999, found that 98,000 people a year are killed by preventable hospital errors. As the eighth cause of death in the United States, medical mistakes cause more deaths than auto accidents. A recent case made headlines when a young girl died who received the wrong organ in a transplant operation because twelve hospital workers and doctors failed to check her blood type.

Study after study reveals serious problems. One out of every twenty-five patients suffers complications from treatment rather than illness, in most cases involving prescription drugs. One in five patients who died in a renowned, state-of-the-art medical center in the Midwest were misdiagnosed. Many health experts estimate that 20–30% of medical procedures are wrongly prescribed.

Fewer than 50% of Medicare patients who suffer heart attacks get the proper drugs, and almost 90% of pharmaceutical errors involve dispensing the wrong drug or dose. One pharmacist was recently jailed by federal prosecutors for diluting drugs used to treat chemotherapy patients for more

Assume An Active Role

than ten years. The use of drugs such as Ritalin to treat children has increased 300–600% in ten years and is attributed to the fact that drugs are cheaper than therapy and are also covered by insurance.

Since 1997, more than a dozen pharmaceutical drugs have been removed from the market by the Food and Drug Administration because they were determined to be unsafe. With over 300,000 adverse reactions reported annually, there are also concerns about the safety of many other drugs, raising serious questions about the FDA's approval process and whether it is too close to the industry it regulates.

Not surprisingly, the Institute of Medicine, which conducted many of the studies cited above, concluded that our health care system is "disjointed and inefficient." These alarming figures point the finger at all health professionals. But they do not take into account mistakes commonly made by consumers, such as taking the wrong dosage of medicine, failing to comply with appropriate medical advice and recommendations, and ignoring a health issue until it becomes more serious or even fatal.

People who have anything to do with our health care system for an extended period of time become one of two types—*health care advocates* or *those who want to become health care advocates*. Assuming an active role in health care is necessary for our survival.

Discard the Old Role

This guide uses the term health care *consumer* in place of *patient*. Although this change in terminology seems superficial on the surface, it is profound in practice.

The role of patient suggests that you are more a bystander than a participant in the health care process. As patients in our health care system, we develop a "Stepford Wife"—type personality, allowing others to make decisions and dictate what is best for us as though we are small children and not able to determine our own needs. This is the health care of the past. The role of consumer signals that you are a full participant in the health process and empowered to make decisions regarding your own care. This is the health care of the future.

The indecipherability of medical technology and terminology serves to empower the people who provide treatment over those who receive it. This limits our participation in the health care process because the average person is not able to understand its complexities. In order to reclaim our power in health care, we must begin to think of ourselves as something other than unknowledgeable patients and helpless victims of our bodies at the mercy of an all-knowing, all-powerful medical establishment, conventional or alternative.

Health care is a business like any other, so as consumers of health care, you should regard your role no differently from your role in purchasing any product or service. If you would not buy a house or car without ensuring that it is what you want and need, why would you buy a health care service without doing the same? You have an absolute right and a responsibility to make sure that you receive the service that is represented to you and that you are not being harmed in any way. The only real danger in assuming a more active role lies in the threat it poses to the autonomy of those in the medical profession.

Patient passivity and submissiveness are still encouraged and often demanded of us by health care professionals. In

Assume An Active Role

fact, they have even given it a clinical name, *patient compliance*, and medical research contains numerous studies on how to increase and encourage it. Today, the benefits of patient compliance in such a troubled health care system are few, hurting us far more than helping us. Assuming an active role in health care promotes the opposite of passivity and submissiveness, but you can assume this role and continue to respect and utilize the opinions and recommendations of others.

Redefining your role in the health care relationship will redefine your role in the health care process, and you will automatically become a better consumer with this realization. Redefining your role also requires an understanding and awareness of the larger picture of health.

People are not powerless to change their health, an old myth still perpetuated in many medical circles. The notion that disease or illness is a phenomenon over which you have little or no control is simply untrue. Providers and medicine are not the source of healing but only facilitate our own natural capacity to heal.

Disease or illness is often a symptom of a much larger issue, which gives it great import. Sometimes, the meaning of illness cannot be derived from physical recovery but from the opportunity to make other changes in our lives.

Adopt a New Role

As a consumer rather than a patient, assuming an active role involves a willingness to acquire the knowledge, attitudes, and behaviors necessary to get the most out of health care. It includes finding the right provider for your needs and changing providers when the relationship no longer benefits you. Providers provide a service, and in most cases, you can choose to use their service or not. This role also demands that you prepare for health care appointments in order to maximize the benefits of visits and are more assertive with providers when it comes to meeting your health needs.

Assuming an active role includes researching health issues and investigating treatment options. This is now easier than ever before because the Internet has revolutionized access to health information that was previously only available to providers.

Engaging in appropriate self-care is another aspect of taking an active role in health care. Proper medication use is no longer the primary self-care issue in health care. Prevention is the primary concern of self-care due to increased environmental threats to our health and well-being.

Communication is the cornerstone of any productive health care relationship, but providers are frequently inaccessible to people either in or out of their offices. Nurses, nurse practitioners, physician assistants, and other medical staff members serve an important function by helping you with your care and treatment, as can other health care consumers.

Consumers have firsthand experience with providers and treatments. They provide the type of uncensored information not available from any other resource. Consumers are particularly helpful in the use of alternative medicine, which is still very much a word-of-mouth business.

You cannot take charge of your health care if you do not know what is happening to you. One of the ways to accomplish this goal is to get copies of medical reports and maintain a copy of your own medical records. Another way to do this is to map your own progress rather than rely solely on the results of diagnostic tests to determine your treatment decisions. A desire to perform these tasks arises from the realization that you possess the knowledge and insight into your own condition that no diagnostic test or medical doctor can possibly have.

In order to take a more active role, an adjustment must be made in your expectations of treatment. Practitioners of alternative medicine have long known that there really is no such phenomenon as the "quick fix" or "magic bullet" in healing. Conventional providers have been slow to accept this fact because there is so much pressure on them to find immediate answers to our problems to alleviate our suffering. Lasting results take time no matter what medicine you use, and you must get used to this reality.

An active role demands that you become familiar with your health care rights. The idea of health care rights is a fairly new concept arising out of a system of medicine that concerns itself with many priorities other than your health. It is also important to be prepared for medical emergencies for all of the obvious reasons. There are several simple things you can do with little effort that will reduce the trauma that arises from an unexpected medical emergency.

Avoid Being a Health Care Victim

Taking precautions to avoid frauds and false claims is an integral part of any comprehensive discussion on assuming an active role in health care. This may be more difficult to accomplish if you have a serious medical condition for which the treatment options are extremely limited.

Health care is especially vulnerable to hucksters and frauds because people who are ill and weak or desperate for answers are easy prey. Unfortunately, there are health care providers who are exploitive, experimental practices of little value, products that are not what they claim to be, and information on the Internet that is misleading or downright untrue.

There are specific signs to alert you to the possibility of bogus health claims. Whenever you see the word "cure," you should exercise extreme caution. Claims of "exclusivity," "miracle remedies," "ancient healing formulas," "incredible results," "scientific breakthroughs," and "government conspiracies" are also causes for concern. You should beware of products or services that are only available to you by advance payment or through foreign clinics.

Take the time to report fraudulent providers to their respective licensing boards and professional associations and fraudulent products to the Federal Trade Commission, Food and Drug Administration, and state Attorney General, Department of Consumer Affairs, or Department of Health.

When you become a more activist and informed health care consumer, you will automatically possess the armor you need to help you avoid becoming a health care victim.

Dealing with Resistence

An empowered consumer represents a shift in the power structure of the health care relationship from a friendly dictatorship to highly collaborative partnership. Providers who

Assume An Active Role

have grown accustomed to the autocratic role they were trained to assume may be reluctant to relinquish this role. They may erroneously believe that your increasing power somehow diminishes theirs.

Consumers who try to take responsibility for their health care are often labeled by providers as "difficult patients." Your empowerment as a health care consumer, however, only increases their ability to help you. *True empowerment can never be diminished but only enhanced by the empowerment of others.*

Although most providers will agree that a proactive consumer is desirable in theory, they may be less comfortable with this concept in practice. This is not true for alternative providers whose clients are actively involved in their own care because the proper application of alternative medicine demands it.

To encourage cooperation from a health care provider, assume an active role on a gradual basis. Remember that providers who resist or discourage your involvement in any way may be practicing medicine for reasons other than your welfare. If this occurs, you may want to find another provider because of the possible negative impact on treatment.

Health care providers who are dedicated to your welfare above all other concerns will welcome the opportunity to join you in a collaborative relationship. Providers understand that they best serve consumers when they are able to step down as medical authorities. Their job becomes easier when they do not have to have all the answers. A collaborative union enhances treatment and improves your chance for a positive outcome—the two benefits that really matter.

Changing Ourselves & Changing the System

An active role advances the notion that you, rather than providers or the system, are in charge of your health and can participate fully in the health care process. It presumes that you are educated about health issues, have the ability to perform certain functions, and possess a level of self-awareness sufficient to make informed decisions about your own care. Research has shown that even the smallest active role, such as making decisions about when to schedule health care appointments, produces health benefits.

As consumers, we can make decisions for ourselves. We can question the status quo and understand that tradition can be changed if it is illogical, irrational, or harmful to us. We can become knowledgeable by gathering health information and investigating treatment options on our own. We can contest unfair treatment and express concern about treatment that falls below an accepted standard of care. We can even demand a higher standard of care if we choose to do so.

Greater power in the health care process leads to greater change in the health care system. Our use of alternative medicine exemplifies this. Despite dire warnings from the conventional medical establishment, consumers have continued to use alternative medicine to compensate for the inadequacies of standard care. More and more people are seeking the advice of alternative providers and using alternative remedies and herbs.

Our use of alternative medicine has grown to the point at which it generates billions of dollars every year. This buying power has motivated an entrenched medical establishment to bend to our will, however begrudgingly, by trying to adopt a more holistic focus and making alternative methods and techniques the subjects of research studies.

Anthropologist Margaret Mead said, "Never doubt that a small group of committed people can change the world." The economic power we wield as consumers is formidable and can effect positive change in our health care system because alternative medicine is now a business like any other in which huge profits are at stake. We must be discriminating in this pursuit, approaching alternative medicine as we would any other service or product—with caution, care, and as much information as possible—a caveat that applies equally to conventional medicine.

3

Are You a Health Care Victim?

Another important aspect to surviving our health care system is to approach it with a sense of humor. The fun, easy quiz that follows was designed to help you rate your status as an active health care consumer. Please note that the results of this quiz are not scientific.

Choose the answer that best applies to you:

1. I choose a health care provider by:
    - ___ a. picking one out of the telephone book.
    - ___ b. going to the first provider affiliated with my health insurance plan.
    - ___ c. getting recommendations from people I trust.
    - ___ d. I don't choose a provider until I get sick.

2. I exercise:
    ___ a. never.
    ___ b. occasionally.
    ___ c. frequently.
    ___ d. every day.

3. When my health insurer unfairly denies a benefit, I:
    ___ a. file an appeal with my insurer.
    ___ b. let it go and do nothing.
    ___ c. call my insurer to complain.
    ___ d. complain to others.

4. If a provider dismisses my questions, I:
    ___ a. do nothing.
    ___ b. persist on getting an answer.
    ___ c. complain to others.
    ___ d. change providers.

5. If a provider makes an honest mistake with my care, I:
    ___ a. tell him about it and ask him to make it right.
    ___ b. change providers.
    ___ c. complain to a professional association or licensing board.
    ___ d. do nothing.

6. If a doctor tells me I need a surgical procedure, I:
    ___ a. take the doctor's word for it and go ahead with the procedure.
    ___ b. do nothing.
    ___ c. get recommendations from family or friends.
    ___ d. get a second opinion.

Are You a Health Care Victim?

7. If a provider is significantly late for an appointment, he should:
   ___ a. do nothing.
   ___ b. apologize for his lateness.
   ___ c. extend the appointment time or reduce his fee.
   ___ d. have his staff handle the problem.

8. If a provider is negative with me, I:
   ___ a. ask him to be more positive or change providers.
   ___ b. do nothing.
   ___ c. complain to the nursing staff.
   ___ d. complain to family and friends.

9. If a provider gives me a hard time about getting copies of my medical records, I:
   ___ a. complain to others.
   ___ b. insist on this right with my provider.
   ___ c. change providers and get copies of records through my new provider.
   ___ d. do nothing.

10. Stress management for me is:
    ___ a. having an alcoholic drink at the end of a day.
    ___ b. taking my frustrations out on others.
    ___ c. taking time to relax every day.
    ___ d. working until the job gets done.

11. If I want to pay up front for a medical service, I:
    ___ a. ask for a cash discount.
    ___ b. pay the full fee without question.

___ c. tell the provider I forgot my checkbook at the end of the appointment.
___ d. complain to others about the cost of the service.

12. I find myself out in nature:
    ___ a. every day.
    ___ b. never.
    ___ c. occasionally.
    ___ d. frequently.

13. I expect a medicine to:
    ___ a. work immediately.
    ___ b. not work at all.
    ___ c. work occasionally.
    ___ d. take time to work.

14. If I have a health care problem, I most want to:
    ___ a. address all elements of the problem.
    ___ b. take a pill to fix it.
    ___ c. ignore the problem.
    ___ d. complain to others.

15. If I have a medical emergency in the future, I:
    ___ a. will let others in charge make decisions for me.
    ___ b. will play it by ear and make decisions as they arise.
    ___ c. will do nothing.
    ___ d. have a health care directive and designated advocate.

Are You a Health Care Victim?

16. Before I go to a health care appointment, I:
    ___ a. do nothing.
    ___ b. wait until the appointment to decide what to say.
    ___ c. take notes and write out questions in advance.
    ___ d. think a little about what I want to say.

17. If I have a health care problem, I prefer to:
    ___ a. rely on my provider for information.
    ___ b. rely on others for information.
    ___ c. do nothing.
    ___ d. research the problem myself.

18. I watch what I eat:
    ___ a. frequently.
    ___ b. occasionally.
    ___ c. never.
    ___ d. every day.

19. I connect with support staff in a provider's office:
    ___ a. frequently.
    ___ b. never.
    ___ c. always.
    ___ d. only when there is a problem.

20. When I receive treatment for a health care problem, I:
    ___ a. ignore it with the hope that it will go away.
    ___ b. do nothing.
    ___ c. depend on others to monitor my progress.
    ___ d. monitor my own progress.

21. I am aware of environmental influences on health:
    ___ a. always.
    ___ b. never.
    ___ c. occasionally.
    ___ d. frequently.

22. Pick the statement that best applies to you:
    ___ a. I know little about my health care rights but would like to learn more.
    ___ b. I am not interested or do not have time to learn about my health care rights.
    ___ c. I prefer to leave health care rights to others.
    ___ d. I know my health care rights.

23. An advance health care directive is primarily:
    ___ a. hospital discharge instructions.
    ___ b. permission to do medical surgery.
    ___ c. instruction on prolonging life with medical intervention.
    ___ d. informed consent for medical care.

24. If all appeals with an insurer have been exhausted for a benefit I still feel entitled to, I:
    ___ a. ask for help from the state agency that monitors insurance activity.
    ___ b. do nothing.
    ___ c. expect the provider to reverse the charge.
    ___ d. complain to others.

25. I have power as a health care consumer to receive the best possible care:
    ___ a. sometimes.

Are You a Health Care Victim?

___ b. always.
___ c. frequently.
___ d. never.

SCORE:

Add up your score into a total number of points and consult the results on the following page.

1.	a=2,	b=3,	c=4,	d=1	_____
2.	a=1,	b=2,	c=3,	d=4	_____
3.	a=4,	b=1,	c=3,	d=2	_____
4.	a=1,	b=4,	c=2,	d=3	_____
5.	a=4,	b=3,	c=2,	d=1	_____
6.	a=2,	b=1,	c=3,	d=4	_____
7.	a=1,	b=3,	c=4,	d=2	_____
8.	a=4,	b=1,	c=3,	d=2	_____
9.	a=2,	b=4,	c=3,	d=1	_____
10.	a=1,	b=2,	c=4,	d=3	_____
11.	a=4,	b=1,	c=2,	d=3	_____
12.	a=4,	b=1,	c=2,	d=3	_____
13.	a=1,	b=2,	c=3,	d=4	_____
14.	a=4,	b=3,	c=1,	d=2	_____
15.	a=2,	b=3,	c=1,	d=4	_____
16.	a=1,	b=2,	c=4,	d=3	_____
17.	a=2,	b=3,	c=1,	d=4	_____
18.	a=3,	b=2,	c=1,	d=4	_____
19.	a=2,	b=1,	c=4,	d=3	_____
20.	a=2,	b=1,	c=3,	d=4	_____
21.	a=4,	b=1,	c=2,	d=3	_____
22.	a=3,	b=1,	c=2,	d=4	_____
23.	a=1,	b=2,	c=4,	d=3	_____
24.	a=4,	b=1,	c=3,	d=2	_____
25.	a=2,	b=4,	c=3,	d=1	_____
				Total	_____

Results:

100 Points = Excellent—You already are an excellent health care consumer! Read this book to reinforce your skills, and then give it to a friend.

75–99 Points = Good—You are a good health care consumer but could improve your knowledge and abilities.

50–74 Points = Fair—Your knowledge and ability as a health care consumer is seriously deficient. You need a lot of improving.

Below 50 Points = Poor—You have health care victim written all over you. Read this book twice!

4

Be Selective About Providers

The first step in assuming an active role in health care is to exercise discernment in choosing providers. They come in all shapes, sizes, and levels of skill, experience, and knowledge. They also have different competencies, attitudes, motivations, and intentions.

It is becoming more and more difficult to find providers who are willing to place your interests above all other concerns and whose frustrations with the insurance industry do not spill over into the treatment room. Qualified providers, however, are out there, and there are numerous ways to find them.

A strong, personal recommendation from another consumer is one of the best ways to find a good provider. Asking a health care provider whom he sees rather than whom he recommends is another way to find a good provider. When it comes to your health, it pays to shop around.

The right to choose your own provider is a hotly debated issue with consumers right now because managed care is notorious for unfairly limiting these choices. If you are a member of a health maintenance organization (HMO), you may be limited in your choice of providers, but most health plans, even the managed care ones, will offer you more than one choice. Preferred Provider networks (PPO) typically offer more choices to subscribers than HMOs, but higher premiums are also charged for these plans.

Find out what your provider options are according to your health plan. Decide whether or not you want to go outside of your plan for a provider, and determine what it will cost you to do so.

There are several health care rights we took for granted fifty years ago: the right to consult the provider of your choice, see a medical specialist, get a second opinion, and end a relationship with a provider. Ironically, consumers are having to fight for these same rights today, which is why Congress has tried to expand the choices of HMO subscribers by passing a comprehensive Patient Bill of Rights.

It is one thing to choose on your own to remain with a provider or see a specialist but quite another to have a third party with no medical training or knowledge of you make this decision for you. Almost one-half of the states have *any willing provider* laws, requiring managed care and insurance networks to accept out-of-network providers as long as the provider accepts the insurer's rate and contract terms.

Health care providers cover many disciplines and practices. They include medical doctors, dentists, optometrists, podiatrists, osteopaths, psychotherapists, urgent care centers, ambulatory surgery centers, hospitals, and surgical teams. They also include nurses, physician assistants, alternative medicine practitioners, pharmacy prescription centers, laboratory technicians, ambulance services, and many others. Any person who provides you with a health service is a health care provider. Remember that you can be just as selective about choosing a hospital or a medical laboratory as you can about choosing a treating physician.

Alternative Medicine

Choosing an alternative provider can be both more easy and more difficult than choosing a conventional provider. Insurance companies do not pay benefits for alternative practices that are not widely taught in medical schools or generally used in hospitals. Benefits are typically paid for chiropractic medicine, osteopathic medicine, and alternative practices that are performed by a medical doctor. Some insurance plans pay benefits for massage if performed by a participating therapist or when prescribed by a medical doctor.

Since most of the costs for alternative medicine come directly out of your pocket, you can change providers at will. There is absolutely no reason why you should be stuck in an unsatisfactory relationship with an alternative provider.

Although there are many alternative providers in metropolitan areas and large towns, there may be few or no alternative providers in small communities. Shopping around for an alternative provider can also be costly because you are responsible for the full fee. There are significant variations among alternative practices and between providers of the same alternative practice. For example, you can talk with several acupuncturists but get a different story from each one of them on what you should do. Doing a fair amount of homework can narrow your search.

Choose an alternative provider who is not only skilled in his field but who is also open to approaches and practices other than his own. An alternative provider like this will be more likely to refer you to another provider if the circumstances warrant.

Investigation

If you are willing to research all your provider options, you can reduce the likelihood of making the wrong choice. Begin by verifying the provider's credentials. Request a copy of his curriculum vitae (CV), which lists his training and experience. Confirm the provider's completion of medical school and residency (or alternative medicine training program). Most doctors complete three years of post-graduate training in an approved residency program. Fellowships provide advanced training in a specialty.

Check the provider's membership status with professional associations, and ensure that his license to practice is current and in good standing with the state medical board. Medical boards also have information about malpractice claims and limitations on clinical privileges. Professional associations will sometimes release information about complaints, but keep in mind that they, along with local medical societies, are not selective about members. No medical authority will tell you about investigations in progress, nor

Be Selective About Providers

can it confirm the competency of providers. (See Appendices A and C.)

Make sure the provider is board certified as a specialist in his field, which means that he has completed an approved residency and passed the board's exam. The American Board of Medical Specialties at (866) 275–2267 or online at www.abms.org recognizes 24 specialities, including internal medicine and family practice. Also, confirm that the provider has hospital privileges or that he is able to admit you to one if it becomes necessary.

Find out more about the provider's practice. When did he graduate from medical school and complete his residency? In conventional medicine, an older provider has more experience, but a younger one has received the latest training. In alternative medicine, experience is what matters the most because the established therapies rarely change. How many days a week does the provider practice, how many clients does he actually see in a week, and how many times has he performed the treatment or procedure you are interested in receiving? Ask around to see if anyone you know has been treated by the provider. Find out if he accepts insurance or other forms of payment like Workers' Compensation and if he participates in the network of your health plan.

Many providers hold professorial positions in medical schools. Full-time professors are on the cutting edge of new technology and have many colleagues at their immediate disposal because they also teach and conduct research. Part-time or "clinical" professors are usually full-time clinicians who perform a limited role in medical schools.

Do not assume that a provider who is well known or the director of a school, department, clinic, or hospital is always the best choice. Although there are exceptions to the rule, providers who serve major administrative or academic roles, become media personalities, or regularly publish books may practice medicine infrequently.

If you can, contact health care providers *before* deciding to use their services because what they do in their respective practices and how they treat you varies greatly. You cannot ask too many questions of a provider because what you do not know about him can definitely hurt you. We have all heard about people who have been caught practicing medicine with no license or the proper training. Unnecessarily or incompetently performed surgeries and procedures have become an all too common thread in the health care tapestry.

Medical doctors have also been known to have substance abuse problems. One well-known plastic surgeon failed to disclose an unresolved drug rehabilitation history to patients and continued to be named among the best doctors in America, despite being sued numerous times for medical malpractice, the latter of which was significant in and of itself. Although you cannot realistically ask a provider for a urine specimen to test for drugs, you can do your homework in advance to reduce the possibility of making a serious mistake.

An important source of information about health care providers is the *National Practitioner's Data Bank* (NPDB), which was created in 1990. The NPDB is operated by the U.S. Health and Human Services' Division of Quality Assurances and was designed to foster more effective communication on provider monitoring.

Every medical malpractice payment that is made by a provider is listed in the NPDB. Every disciplinary action taken against a provider by a state licensing board, hospital,

Be Selective About Providers

professional association, malpractice insurer, and the U.S. Drug Enforcement Agency is also listed in the NPDB.

The creation of this online data bank has had two important repercussions. It discourages providers from settling legitimate malpractice claims with consumers because they do not want to be listed in the NPDB. It has also created an outcry from provider organizations, which claim that the NPDB unfairly tarnishes the reputation of members who settle frivolous malpractice cases just to get rid of them. These organizations also contend that the NPDB discourages the overall settlement of claims.

An online data bank such as the NPDB is only helpful to the extent that all complaints against providers are fairly and impartially heard and that appropriate disciplinary sanctions are imposed by the relevant parties. Unfortunately, too many bad providers are able to slip through the cracks of a system that continues to be stacked in their favor.

Data from the NPDB is currently only available to hospitals, managed care organizations, licensing boards, professional associations, and other health care groups, although there are efforts afoot to make it directly available to consumers. Until then, you may be able to get the information from someone who has access to the NPDB, or you can be bold and ask the provider yourself if he is listed in the NPDB. His failure to answer may suggest that he has made a medical malpractice payment or has had a disciplinary action taken against him, alerting you to the need for further investigation.

There are other sources of information on bad providers. State medical licensing boards provide information on disciplinary actions for a small fee, and many provide information on medical malpractice judgments. The "civil index" of the County or Superior Court Clerk's office maintains a list of lawsuits that have been filed against a provider. This is important information for consumers, particularly in the presence of multiple malpractice complaints. Multiple complaints filed against a provider cannot be collectively dismissed as frivolous regardless of their outcomes. At the very least, they suggest that the provider has a serious communication problem with his clients.

There are several online services that provide information about doctors, but beware of those that receive fees from doctors, hospitals, and insurers for the obvious reasons. An online databank of disciplinary actions at www.questionabledoctors.org provides information on disciplinary actions taken by 27 state licensing boards and federal agencies such as the U.S. Department of Health and Human Services, Drug Enforcement Administration, and Food and Drug Administration. Reports are available for only a specified time period and for a slightly higher fee than charged by government agencies. Other fee-based services are available at www.healthgrades.com and www.docinfo.org.

Information about health care organizations is provided by the Joint Commission on Accreditation of Healthcare Organizations (JCAHO) at (603) 792–5000 or online at www.jcaho.org. This is an independent, nonprofit agency that evaluates and accredits almost 20,000 health care organizations including hospitals, HMO's, health networks, and other health-oriented groups. Call hospitals in advance to find out what services they provide, their costs and payment plans, and their ability to accommodate special needs. Find out if the hospital employs a patient safety officer who is responsible for overseeing the management of medical errors. (See Chapter 15.)

It is a good idea to contact medical laboratories in advance of using their services because they can differ significantly in their charges for the same diagnostic tests. Some laboratories offer cash discounts and, with proper authorization, will send copies of test results directly to consumers.

Pharmacy prescription centers can be consulted about their prices, special discounts, and mail or delivery service. Some pharmacies will contact doctors directly on your behalf to renew or make changes to your prescription medications. If you want to purchase prescription drugs from an online pharmacy, make sure that it is licensed and the drugs are as advertised.

Introductory Consultations

If you can afford to do so, consult with more than one provider before selecting one. Introductory consultations can assist you in this effort. They are brief, "get-to-know-you" office visits, lasting anywhere from five to fifteen minutes. These consults are educational and informative, giving you the opportunity to meet the provider with no obligation to receive treatment from him or see him again. Costs for introductory consultations differ, but should be significantly less than the cost of a normal office visit.

Without introductory consultations, interviewing more than one provider before choosing one may not be very practical. Initial consultations for both conventional and alternative providers tend to be lengthy and expensive. Interviewing more than one conventional provider is only possible if you have a small copayment with your insurance plan for physician consultations.

Consultations with alternative providers can be even more cost-prohibitive. For example, initial visits with a homeopathic doctor typically last two hours at a cost of $250 or more. Despite this, alternative providers are usually more inclined than their conventional counterparts to agree to introductory consultations at little or no cost to you.

Before meeting with a provider for the first time, prepare a list of questions you want to ask and take it with you to the appointment. You can include questions about the provider's background, experience, and success in treating people with your condition. Find out what methods and techniques he specializes in, how his approach differs from others, and what he expects from you. You also need to know how to communicate with him outside the appointment time and what his policies are on fees and billing.

What to Look For

There are several criteria you should take into account when selecting a health care provider. You must consider a provider's: *skill*, which takes into account his knowledge, training, education, experience, and natural ability; *intention*, which is his motivation for practice; and *compatibility*, which is how well you get along and communicate with him and the congruency of goals for the relationship and treatment. For example, a provider who does not want consumers to manage their own care will not be a good match for the person who seeks more authority to do so.

Be Selective About Providers

You gain knowledge about a provider's training and experience through his curriculum vitae and can discover how compatible you are with him in an introductory consultation. But you can only determine his natural ability and motivation for practice with firsthand treatment experience, which is revealed over time as your condition improves or worsens.

Recommendations from consumers you know and trust will help you initially decide with whom to consult, but health care experiences vary enormously from person to person and condition to condition. What is helpful to one person may be harmful to another. For example, deep tissue massage may be relaxing to one person but excruciatingly painful to another. Only you can ultimately decide the right provider for you.

Intention

It is important to be aware of the extent to which intention or motivation affects your care and treatment. Intentions that exclude your welfare complicate health care relationships and interfere with treatment process and outcome. This is not an issue commonly discussed in medical circles because doctors do not like to admit that they have motives other than helping you to get well. Since the repercussions can be serious, a provider's intention should always be considered in the selection process.

People are motived to enter the health care field for many reasons, including a desire to help people, contribute to society, facilitate health, and give back to others. They also do it out of a desire for money, notoriety, control, importance, and to compete with others. Obviously, you want to choose health care providers whose intentions are the former rather than the latter—those who care more about serving you than serving themselves. Providers should place the quality of your care above all other concerns.

Everyone knows at least one health care provider who suffers from the malady known as the "doctor syndrome." In this pathological state, the provider has delusions that his power exists in the initials that follow his name, leading to chronic symptoms of imperiousness and arrogance. Although this syndrome is usually associated with medical doctors, it applies to other health providers as well. As we all know, power does not emanate from having a degree but from what one does with the degree. It is about what the provider stands for and who he is as a person as well as a healer.

We should not be surprised that there are providers who are focused more on themselves than on their clients because of our societal emphasis on individual achievement and material success. Basic medical school criteria for becoming a doctor are good grades, the stamina to survive medical training, and the money to pay for it. Many people become doctors for the status, prestige, and high incomes that are expected to follow.

Health care providers must have a clear understanding of their role in your treatment and care in order to truly help you. Our Western approach to medicine includes a belief that the doctor is responsible for making you well. This is a gross misrepresentation of the role that he plays. Providers do not heal but merely facilitate healing.

Health care providers who believe they are the source of healing set themselves up for inevitable failure and you for disappointment along with possible harm. Remember that you can be hurt as much by a provider's intent as you can their lack of skill.

Compatibility

You must find a health care provider with whom you are compatible. Research that examines patient satisfaction with treatment outcome strongly suggests that the quality of the health care relationship is as important as, if not more important than, the treatment itself. We need to pay close attention to this. Since communication is the foundation for any successful relationship, you must be able to communicate well with your provider in order to ensure a positive outcome from treatment.

Providers should be willing and able to talk with you about any aspect of health—physical, psychological, and spiritual. What is his communication style? Is he respectful, helpful, positive, supportive, easy to understand, and a good listener?

Avoid providers who make you feel uneasy about or are dismissive toward your needs and concerns, especially the ones that are embarrassing to you. In health care relationships, you should feel truly and deeply heard by a provider who should also be able to consistently and positively respond to your expressed needs.

Extremism and inflexibility are also red flags when it comes to choosing health care providers. If providers are stuck in beliefs that are in conflict with your needs or are immoderate in their approach to treatment, their ability to help you will be seriously compromised.

Conservatism

The opposite of extremism is conservatism, an attribute frequently overlooked in a crisis-focused health care system but another important criterion in choosing a health care provider. Remember the phrase "everything in moderation"?

Providers who are conservative make realistic claims about achievable results, reducing the possibility for medical error and harm. They are also willing to take the time necessary to find the right treatment for your condition. Conservatism is especially important in the use of alternative medicine, in which ridiculous claims are often made about what can be accomplished.

Most health care providers can only recommend the medicine they are trained to use because of medical specialization and an absence of collaboration between and within the conventional and alternative systems of medicine. As a result of this, conventional providers tend to apply crisis treatment to noncrisis conditions, and alternative providers apply noncrisis treatment to crisis conditions. Providers who are conservative know the difference between these two approaches and the one that is right for you. Providers like these will refer you elsewhere if they cannot help you.

Fees for Service

If you do not have health insurance, a provider is not covered by your plan, or you choose to pay up front for a service, you should *always* ask for a cash discount. Requesting it in advance of treatment gives you more negotiating power

Be Selective About Providers

because the provider knows you can always seek treatment elsewhere. Cash discounts should be available for any conventional service that is normally eligible for insurance benefits. Sometimes, you have to pay in actual cash, rather than by check or credit card, in order to get a cash discount.

Conventional providers tend to be inflexible about fees, so be prepared for cash discounts that are not very sizable. The typical cash discount for a conventional provider is 10% off their usual fee. For a fee of $120, this is only $12, which is hardly equitable if the provider has already agreed to accept $75 from an insurer for the same service and only after filing extensive paperwork. At the very least, a provider should be willing to accept the same amount from you that he has agreed to receive from the insurer because you are saving him the time and expense of all the paperwork.

Although you will probably have to ask for cash discounts from conventional providers, alternative providers may offer them to you without your having to ask. Alternative medicine fees are lower to begin with; an alternative provider may charge $75 or less for the same amount of treatment time for which the conventional provider charges $120. Depending on the practice, alternative providers may also provide a discount for a series of treatments.

Realistic Expectations

Be selective about providers, but also have realistic expectations of them. They are not perfect and require the same understanding and tolerance you would afford any important relationship. Decide for yourself what qualities are necessary in a provider, and be willing to compromise on what is not, as long as you can perform an active role and have a reasonable expectation that your health needs are being met. The bottom line is that you want to get the most from your health care with the least number of risks and inconveniences. In an imperfect world with an imperfect system, you must balance your needs with the provider's abilities.

Forget television's *Marcus Welby M.D.* or the doting doctors from *ER*. There is a huge gap between how the medical profession is portrayed publicly and how it plays out in real life. Once upon a time, doctors made house calls when you were too sick to go to their office and did not need a six-figure salary to feel good about themselves. The business of medicine has changed all that forever.

Many alternative providers still practice the old, self-sacrificing ways. As alternative medicine becomes incorporated into conventional medicine and its providers adopt the same detached attitudes as their conventional counterparts, the profit motive and gatekeeper mentality of conventional medicine is sure to follow.

Actively involved health care consumers know that good providers place their needs first and encourage responsible, informed health care choices. These providers want collaborative partnerships with consumers rather than autocratic or dictatorial ones. Hierarchical relationships provide only short-term satisfaction, which is eventually replaced with the disappointment that arises from any lopsided alliance. Good providers are willing to participate in equitable partnerships with consumers with the understanding that

Be Selective About Providers

the more involved that consumers are in their own care, the easier that their job is going to be.

☑ Check List
---

1. Get recommendations of health providers from people you know and trust.

2. Gather as much information as possible about providers in advance of meeting them.

3. Request brief, introductory consultations with providers if you want to shop around before making a decision.

4. Evaluate providers on their skill, intention, and compatibility.

5. Seek out providers who make realistic claims and use the right medicine for the right circumstance.

6. Have realistic expectations of providers and what they can do for you.

5

Prepare for Appointments

Few people prepare in advance for health care appointments, but it is a big mistake not to do so. The reason most people think that preparing for health care visits is unnecessary is because they do not believe that they are in charge of their own care. This attitude is a symptom of the *patient syndrome*, which was discussed in the second chapter.

As a *patient*, you do not know what is wrong with you, what caused it, what you need to fix it, or what options are available to you. This is for others to decide. As an educated and informed *consumer*, you know these things or possess the skills necessary to determine them. You will get so much more out of a health care visit by preparing in advance for your appointment.

Advance preparation allows you to maximize the appointment time, allowing you to organize your thoughts and outline your priorities. It forces you to think about what you want to accomplish and what questions you want to ask. It results in greater clarity about your condition and the ability to relay your needs and concerns to your provider more effectively. More efficient use of the appointment time will ultimately translate into lower costs for service and fewer co-payments. Advance preparation is a small price to pay for significantly improved care.

Topics for Discussion

The manner in which you prepare for a health care appointment depends on the service you want to receive, your reasons for seeking treatment, and your expectations and needs. Different health care practices necessitate different forms of preparation.

For example, a visit with a primary care physician would be aided by making a list of general physical symptoms and their effects. For an appointment with a medical specialist, this list would have a more specific focus. Making a list of emotional issues or arranging for a spouse or partner to be with you at a therapy session might facilitate a psychotherapy appointment.

Generally speaking, you prepare for health care visits by composing a list of questions you want to ask and concerns you have regarding your condition and treatment and by taking this list with you to your appointment. Any

Prepare for Appointments

health-related issue, whether it is about your condition, its underlying cause, treatment options, benefits, risks, adverse reactions, and follow-up care, is appropriate for discussion. If you are seeing a new provider, questions about his qualifications to treat you are also relevant.

Your list of topics for discussion should generally include the following:

- the nature of your complaint(s)—symptoms, observances, and concerns

- how the condition affects your life—work, social, and personal—and, conversely, how your life affects the condition

- all options for treatment—benefits, risks, potential outcomes, adverse reactions, and long-term effects

- what type of follow-up care is required—additional appointments, diagnostic tests, additional costs, communication issues, and how your concerns and problems will be handled as they arise

- what you can do to help—self-care issues such as special dietary requirements or physical exercises

- alternative medicine or experimental treatment options that may help your condition

- the provider's willingness to refer you to another provider if he cannot help you

- the prognosis for your condition—full or partial recovery and percentage of permanent change

Write down questions and concerns you want to discuss in order of their importance. Be as succinct and as uncomplicated as possible in your descriptions. Be specific about what you want to know and what you want the provider to do for you. Leave space after each item to write down answers because it is easy to forget what was said by the time you arrive home. In fact, research shows that people remember only 10% of what health providers tell them in appointments. Check off each item on your list as it is addressed to avoid confusion about what has been discussed or omitted because health care visits are often rushed and intimidating.

Know your health history. Obtain a copy of your medical records by sending a signed, written request with the appropriate identifying information to your previous doctor. Providers may charge a fee for copying your records, and it can take several weeks for you or your new provider to receive them.

If time is limited, make a list of the health care treatments you have received and the medications you have taken. Include in your list alternative medicine treatments and remedies you are using to treat your condition. If you wear any appliances or use any products that are related to your condition, bring them with you. Finally, it is important to form realistic expectations about what is going to happen during the appointment.

Alternative Medicine

Preparing for alternative medicine appointments involves more effort because treatment is usually received on the first visit. If you are unfamiliar with the alternative practice, find out what will happen during the first session and what is expected of you afterward.

Sometimes, there are special precautions you need to take prior to an alternative medicine appointment. You may be asked to avoid wearing perfume or nail polish to allow for a more accurate diagnosis. You may also be asked to avoid the consumption of certain foods and alcohol or to engage in a specific exercise or discipline such as meditation or yoga.

Alternative providers will usually devote the beginning of each treatment session to discussion, allowing you more time to express yourself than you would normally be given in a conventional visit. You may also be asked to document your symptoms during treatment and record changes that occur in every aspect of your health—emotional, physical, and spiritual—because they are all part of the alternative medicine assessment.

Other Considerations

Initial appointments obviously necessitate more preparation than follow-up ones because you are not yet familiar with the provider or his practice. For initial appointments, follow the guidelines listed in the previous chapter about selecting a health care provider. Preparation for initial appointments includes evaluating the provider's credentials, talking with others about their treatment experiences, getting previous treatment records, and researching practices and treatment options through various health information sources (see Chapter 7).

Follow-up appointments entail evaluating your progress from treatment, addressing problems and concerns that arise from treatment, and what you and your provider can do to resolve them. At this juncture, it may be helpful to maintain a health diary (see Chapter 12). Issues with the health care relationship, such as difficulties communicating with a provider or his office staff, and issues at work or home that may have an impact on your health can also be addressed. As treatment progresses, questions will also arise about insurance billing and payment.

You may consult with a provider to get a second medical opinion. Second opinions are warranted if you feel uncomfortable with anything a provider has said or done. They are also recommended in the presence of a high risk test or treatment, an unsuccessful treatment, a life-threatening or an uncertain diagnosis, a rare medical condition, medical surgery, or concerns with competence. Since the solicitation of a second medical opinion usually entails a single office visit, be fully prepared for it before you go and make sure that you get all your questions answered.

Health care appointments are filled with many distractions. You cannot make informed choices about your health during an appointment if you do not have all the information you need at your disposal. Advanced preparation is important for this reason.

Like all the steps in this guide, this step is a self-educating one. The more you know about what you want and need, the more you will learn about yourself. The more you know about yourself, the more you can contribute to your own health.

Prepare for Appointments

☑ Check List

1. Preparing for health care appointments takes many forms, depending on the practice, your reasons for seeking treatment, and your individual needs.

2. Find out if there are special requirements for an appointment with a provider, particularly an alternative medicine one.

3. Preparation for appointments generally includes composing a list of questions and concerns about your condition and care, making them as specific and as clear as you can, and taking it with you to the appointment.

4. Initial appointments involve doing research on a provider, his practice, your condition, and treatment options, and follow-up appointments usually have to do with the effects of treatment.

5. Preparation for appointments always includes developing realistic expectations about what will happen during the visit.

6

Assert Yourself with Providers

Becoming an activist health care consumer obliges you to become more assertive in health care relationships. After all, no one has your best interests at heart more than you. Providers have many interests: your health, the welfare of other patients, staying abreast of medical developments, and getting paid. In this relationship, you have only one interest—you!

Medical mistakes and unsafe medical products are simply facts of life. Health providers can be overly decisive, dismissive, and distant. Sometimes, they lack interest in or understanding of all the circumstances affecting your condition. Providers often fail to disclose *all* adverse risks from treatment, making a lack of informed consent a serious and prevalent problem.

You must become more assertive in health care relationships for all of these reasons. Although you cannot eliminate the possibility of harm when you do this, you can significantly reduce its likelihood. This is not the time nor the place to be timid or shy.

Why It Is So Difficult

We forget that medical practice is supposed to be a service industry because its priorities have become so misplaced in recent decades. Health care providers are supposed to serve us, not the other way around. We have also been all too willing to defer health decisions to the expertise of others and are encouraged in this role by those who run the system and by the complexities of a technology-based medicine.

Our powerlessness as health care consumers intimidates us in numerous ways: insurance companies have the power to deny us needed treatment and benefits, providers discern what we should or should not know about our condition and treatment, and the government decides what is legal for both of them to do to us.

Frankly, conventional medical appointments are akin to being run over by a truck. The indifference and abruptness of assembly-line medical service can be stressful and even traumatic, depending on the sensitivity or lack thereof of the provider and his staff. Researchers estimate that the average health visit lasts only 19 minutes, during which time consumers have the opportunity to ask only

Assert Yourself with Providers

four questions, with 23 seconds to set the agenda before the doctor takes over.

Unfortunately, we have become so accustomed to this type of vice-grip service that we rarely consider its impropriety or the harm that it can cause. It would behoove providers to remember that their favorite axiom "Do no harm" applies to our minds as well as our bodies and that words (their presence or absence) can be as injurious to us as a misused scalpel or the wrong drug. How we are treated places our health at risk as much as what we are treated with.

Providers may be insensitive to our needs for many reasons. Some providers were like this long before attending medical school, possessing no social skills or bedside manners. Others have become this way after succumbing to the stresses of medical training and practice. There are also providers who are so taken with themselves that it simply does not occur to them to be kind to the people they serve, particularly if they are successful in their respective practices. Provider insensitivity, depending on how it manifests itself, can be a huge obstacle on the road to health.

Once the appointment is over, your problems may have only just begun. Medical billing services, often based out of town, then assume control. These services are not always cooperative in addressing your concerns or in correcting their mistakes. Meanwhile, their computerized systems continue to spit out monthly bills and, after a specified period of time, will turn even a partially paid account over to a collection agency.

For example, it took one consumer more than one year and, ultimately, the doctor's involvement to get a billing agency to remedy an incorrect date of service for what was then only a $3 copayment. Another billing service sent an insurance claim to the wrong address for months. After a physician's office accepted a reduced amount as payment in full, the billing service continued to demand payment for the difference until the state medical board intervened.

Power lies in medical jargon and with the rarified few who make it their profession. As consumers, this techno-pharmacologically based terminology seems completely beyond our grasp. It is no coincidence that this special language is understood by those who create it rather than those to whom it applies, and it is the rare provider who takes the necessary time to explain it. Alternative medicine, with a seemingly infinite number of treatment options, also complicates our choices rather than simplifies them. This health care environment would be daunting to anyone.

Our medical system has so much power over us that it is easy to feel crushed by it. Detached and expensive, health care is fraught with chaos and disorganization and has the potential for causing us both psychological and physical harm. As result of all this, people usually become assertive with providers only after they have had a bad experience. Although tragedy provides enormous incentive for change, you should not wait to be injured or ill before wanting better health care. You can prevent a bad outcome before it ever happens.

Our complacent approach to health care in the past has created an extremely precarious environment for us today. The consequences of not being assertive in this environment are indeed dire. We have the ability to shift the power from the system to ourselves if we choose to do so. We can demand that the system adapt to our needs rather than the other way around, even in an environment of managed care.

Assert Yourself with Providers

Being assertive with providers takes many different forms and is an attitude as well as a behavior. As an attitude, assertiveness requires inner confidence and strength. As a behavior, it requires the skill to perform it effectively.

Taking Action

Most problems with health providers arise from poor communication. Either you are not making your wishes known to your provider or he is not listening to you. Once you take care of the former, you can be attentive to the latter.

Start at the top of the list you prepared prior to your visit. Raise your greatest concern first, and then follow with your remaining questions. Be honest about bad health habits and willing to speak frankly about any health issue, even those that embarrass you. If a provider is uncomfortable with intimate disclosures, find one who is not.

Expect complete answers to questions, and insist that explanations about your condition and treatment be explained to you in language that you can understand. If you do not understand an answer, ask your provider to explain it to you in simpler terms. If he has no answer, ask him to find it for you. Do not allow a provider to dismiss your concerns or treat you with unwarranted negativity. If you disagree with his recommendations, tell him why.

If you still have questions about treatment after leaving a provider's office, call him. Insist on communicating directly with the provider about important matters, not a nurse or other member of his office staff. Providers who fail to respond to your questions within a day or two or who refuse to communicate with you outside the appointment time if problems arise should be replaced.

Find out what you can do on your own to facilitate treatment. Get the pros and cons about treatment before it is administered or performed, not after it causes an unexpected or unpleasant complication. In conventional medicine, there are always possible complications. If you are presented with difficult treatment choices, ask your provider what he would do if the patient were his spouse or another close family member.

Insist on considering all your treatment options, including experimental and alternative medicine ones. Ask your provider about the availability of generic drugs and any disadvantages in using them over brand name drugs. Immediately alert your provider to treatment outcomes that are undesirable or unexpected.

With so many natural alternatives, prescription drugs should be a last resort instead of the first line of defense. Question providers who advise you to take drugs on an indefinite basis. Sometimes, this is appropriate, but many times, it is not. The purpose of medicine is to encourage your body's own ability to function properly. Taking drugs indefinitely does just the opposite, encouraging dependency along with risking serious side effects and potential long-term consequences.

For a patient with an enlarged prostate, one provider prescribed the drug Flomax indefinitely. The side effects from the use of this drug include back pain, chest pain, headache, dizziness, decreased sex drive, and vertigo. For an arthritic patient, another provider prescribed the drug Plaquenil indefinitely. The side effects from the use of this drug are nausea, skin rash, hair loss, dizziness, and blurred vision, leading to blindness. Both of these clients were savvy enough to use the drugs prescribed for them only temporarily. One replaced the drug with natural remedies, and the other was able to discontinue the drug altogether while continuing to maintain the results.

Write down everything that you can, and do not be afraid to ask a provider to put it in writing. If he is unwilling to commit what he tells you to paper, get a second opinion. This is simply responsible consumerism, which will protect you in the event you are being misled. Any provider who fails to perform a promised service, provides a service below the standard of care for the practice, or puts his needs above your own should be confronted about his behavior with a request that it change.

Be willing to replace a provider if there is no improvement from treatment or if the relationship ceases to be beneficial to you. Since a provider makes more money the longer you seek care, his good intentions are the only incentive he has to resolve your problem expeditiously. This is especially true in the use of alternative medicine. If a provider's actions cause you serious harm, file a complaint against him with the appropriate licensing board and professional association to protect other consumers.

To recapitulate, five things a doctor should never say to you are:

1. *I don't have the time* or any implication that he is too busy to help you.

2. *You can take this drug forever.* There are always side effects from the use of conventional drugs, especially long-term, for which there are usually a variety of natural alternatives.

3. *There are no adverse effects from treatment.* Failure to disclose *all* risks from treatment is a common complaint about the medical profession.

4. *There is nothing you can do to improve your condition.* There are many things you can do, even if your condition is grave.

5. *You will not get better.* No doctor knows this for certain, and many who have made this claim have been proven wrong.

There are also practical matters for you to consider in getting the most from a health care provider. Ask him to communicate with you by email, assuring him that you will only exercise this option when medically necessary. Schedule appointments in the morning when the provider is neither tired nor running late. Insist on the entire time allotted for your appointment, even if he is running late. If the time or cost of an appointment is other than what was represented to you, request an explanation and appropriate adjustment in charges.

Scrutinize your bill and insurance explanation of benefits (EOB) because providers and their billing services can and often do make mistakes. Question unfair or excessive charges, particularly if you are paying a portion or all of them. Expect providers to care more about your welfare than their reimbursement. Finally, insist on understanding and maintaining a copy of your own medical records, and to that end, ask providers to copy you on all diagnostic test results.

Remember to report your use of alternative medicine to your conventional provider and your use of conventional medicine to your alternative provider. The majority of people (more than 60%) do not do the former because they fear a negative response or a lack of knowledge and understanding from their conventional doctors. Their fears are often justified because conventional providers continue to regard alternative medicine with a fair amount of suspicion and disapproval. Failing to disclose your use of other medicines to your provider, however, can be harmful to your health. Medicines can react to one another, causing them to become ineffective, harmful, or even fatal.

Using an Advocate

If you are not naturally assertive and feel uncomfortable in this role, you must find someone else to do it for you. Anyone who knows you well and whom you trust such as a family member or friend, can serve as a health care advocate. Advocates can accompany you to health care appointments and intercede on your behalf when circumstances warrant.

When consulting a medical specialist, your primary care provider can also be an advocate. The advantages of his serving this function are obvious. Since your primary doctor speaks the language and understands the bureaucracy, he can presumably get things done that you might otherwise be unable to accomplish.

Assertive Versus Aggressive

All of the tasks in this guide require assertiveness on some level, but this task will probably elicit the most resistance from health professionals. It also has the greatest potential for confrontation. Assertiveness can be as benign as asking for answers to questions, but it can also be as difficult as having to confront a provider about harmful attitudes or actions.

The manner in which you assert yourself with providers will determine the outcome. Developing good communication skills is essential in this process because it teaches you the difference between being assertive and being aggressive.

Assertiveness involves expressing your needs and wants and taking personal responsibility for your feelings at the same time. This is accomplished in such a way that the listener is disinclined to become hostile or defensive. You can demonstrate to the provider that your demands are reasonable and flexible, cooperating with him within acceptable parameters. When you are assertive, you always show consideration for the other person's feelings. An assertive approach is characterized by "I" statements, such as "I feel this way because . . . " or "I would appreciate it if you would. . . ."

Aggressiveness involves initiating personal attacks without consideration for the listener's feelings, making unreasonable demands, or being noncompliant without cause. An aggressive approach includes "You" statements, such as "You did this to me" or "You have to do this or else." An aggressive approach only serves to antagonize and alienate the provider, cornering him with blame and leaving him without any possible exit. An aggressive approach does not allow the provider to alter his view or change his behavior without being humiliated or shamed.

One of the keys to the success of this approach is having your provider regard you more as a consumer than a patient. One study suggested that the sicker people are, the

Assert Yourself with Providers

more physicians regard them as patients, and the healthier people are, the more they regard them as customers. This translates into horizontal, or lying down, equals patient and vertical, or standing upright, equals customer. Medical doctors know how to treat patients, but many of them do not know how to treat customers. It is up to you to change this dynamic.

Being assertive with providers represents a dramatic change in the power structure of the health care relationship, and this change is definitely to your advantage. The extent to which you want to be assertive depends on what you need and how badly you need it.

You are entitled to have a productive, beneficial health care relationship, and your provider is obliged to ensure this, unless your demands are unreasonable or potentially harmful to your health. When you become assertive with a provider, you take a giant leap in ensuring the best possible care, and better care results in better treatment outcomes.

☑ Check List

1. Learn to assert yourself with health care providers before you become ill or have a bad experience.

2. Insist on good communication about all aspects of health in and outside of scheduled appointment times.

3. Request all the information at the provider's disposal, and demand understandable explanations about your condition and treatment including all possible outcomes and risks before they occur.

4. Do not be afraid to ask for what you want, and do not be afraid to ask for it in writing.

5. Be prepared to replace a provider or file a complaint if the service provided falls below the standard of care for the practice.

6. Use an advocate if you have difficulty being assertive in health care relationships.

7

Do Your Own Research

A responsible consumer who uses medicine wisely is a consumer who does not merely take the word of another without his or her own investigation. Be willing to research health issues on your own. Once you have found the right provider and have developed a good relationship with him, you can then focus on gathering as much information as possible about your condition.

There is a positive and negative side to researching health issues. Health information is more accessible to the public than ever before, but there is so much of it that it can be overwhelming. Thanks to the Information Age, there may be such a phenomenon as "too much information."

Health information is also complex because it involves medical terminology, which, as we know, is like a foreign language. It can also be contradictory because medical research is in a constant state of flux, changing its mind with each new study. One study finds a positive effect from a treatment, and another finds a negative one or no effect at all. For example, antibiotics are beneficial, but now they are harmful if used on a chronic basis. Also, health professionals do not always agree with one another. You should research health issues on your own to the extent that it alleviates your confusion but does not contribute to it.

Be extremely discerning about the sources of information you use. Ask your provider for his recommendations, and use common sense and good judgment when researching health information.

Consumer Resources

There are many sources of health information on health conditions, medical drugs, herbal remedies, diagnostic tests, self-care issues, surgical procedures, experimental treatments, and alternative medicine practices. Remember that you must verify the reliability of the source before using the information.

Common sources of health information include the following:

- consumers
- health care providers
- public, university, and health science libraries

Do Your Own Research

- health information research services
- federal and state agencies
- practice organizations and associations
- consumer and medical advocacy groups
- hospital programs
- medical support groups
- medical schools and training programs
- medical pharmacies
- local and national media
- Internet
- bookstores
- natural health retail businesses

The Internet

The Internet has created an information revolution, and one of its greatest contributions is making health information readily available to the public. Information that was previously the domain of health professionals is now just a mouse click away. Surfing the Internet can also be extremely frustrating and time-consuming if you do not know exactly what information you need or where to find it.

It is estimated that approximately 17 million people use the Internet to access health information. There are many online resources for consumers through search engines like Google, Yahoo, MSN, and Infoseek.

Most libraries have large computer databases, which you can search from your home computer by connecting with their Internet website. If you do not have a home computer, most public libraries offer free Internet access on theirs. Library databases allow you access to books, book chapters, trade and consumer magazines, academic journals, newspaper articles, government publications, audiovisual materials (films and videotapes), sound recordings, and scientific research.

Many periodicals and medical journals have their own websites, allowing you direct access to articles and archives for a fee. Government health agencies, consumer advocacy groups, and professional associations for conventional and alternative medicine also have websites. You can connect with other consumers about health issues on the Internet through chatrooms, discussion groups, and message boards.

Some Internet sites for researching general health issues include:

Aetna™/ Harvard Medical School
www.intelihealth.com

Blue Shield of California
www.mylifepath.com

Health On the Net Foundation
www.hon.ch

Karolinska Institute
www.mic.ki.se/Diseases

Mayo Clinic
www.mayohealth.org

Medscape/WebMD
www.medscape.com

Do Your Own Research

National Network of Libraries of Medicine
  (Greater Midwest Region)
  healthweb.org

University of Cincinnati/Ohio State University/
  Case Western Reserve
  www.netwellness.org

You must be extremely selective about health information on the Internet because the quality of information on the Internet varies greatly, in part because virtually anyone can have a website. It is estimated that 70% of all health information found on the Internet is false or misleading. Medical advice from cyberspace should never be substituted for medical advice from a qualified health care provider.

Restrict yourself to sites sponsored by established medical centers, universities, and government agencies. Always consider the source of the information before you use it. When in doubt, confirm the information with at least two other reliable sources before assuming it is true.

Internet sites that provide health information should clearly identify themselves and their qualifications and fully disclose their purpose or mission. If you cannot determine who they are, who funds them, or what their purpose is, seek information elsewhere.

Some sites begin by offering you health information but are really designed to sell products, in which case the information is likely slanted to promote their sale. Some websites do not sell products per se but receive a fee for products sold by other companies that are featured on the site.

The best defense in protecting yourself against bad information on the Internet is to employ simple common sense. Are the claims realistic? It may be logical that fatigue can be reduced by cleansing the digestive tract, but does it make sense that an exclusive diet of sprouts will cure cancer?

There are literally thousands of websites on alternative medicine. Many of them come and go with lightning speed. There is less scientific data on alternative medicine to confirm the claims that are made, so you should exercise the same caution, if not more, when researching alternative treatments. Keep in mind that alternative medicine is highly individualized, and what works for one person may not work for another.

The Federal Trade Commission (FTC) monitors Internet health sites for fraud and misinformation and maintains a listing of recommended health websites at www.ftc.gov. Other rating services, such as Health On the Net and Health Summit Working Group, also provide their own lists of recommended sites.

A group based at the University of Oxford in England has developed a questionnaire, which is available online at www.discern.org.uk, to help consumers assess the quality of online health information. Websites that display the "HONcode" logo from Health On the Net are required to follow certain principles of honesty, confidentiality, and disclosure, and websites displaying the "TRUSTe" seal follow specific guidelines to protect your privacy.

In the future, the Internet is expected to become even more important in health care. More than half of the people in the United States will soon have disposable income, college educations, and computers. The demand for information is high and consumer driven. Along with providing health information, the Internet will be increasingly used for health care support, consumer-provider communication, provider information, and electronic medical records.

Internet programs such as Life Masters® already provide online health monitoring for the elderly and people with chronic disease. Not only do programs like this make health care more cost-effective, but they also provide people with regular care.

Medical Information Services

The Internet has generated a number of medical information services that research health topics for a fee, which varies considerably from service to service. You can also contact the National Health Information Center at (800) 336–4797 for referrals to federal and private organizations that provide information on specific diseases.

Fee-based information services include:

Can Help (360) 437–2291
Health Resource (800) 949–0090 or (501) 329–5272
Medical Information Foundation (800) 999–1999 or
 (650) 326–6000
Planetree Foundation (415) 923–3680.
Schine Online Services (800) 346–3287 or
 (401) 751–3320
World Research Foundation (928) 284–3300

To research prescription medications, consult the *Physician's Drug Resource* (PDR) at your provider's office or local pharmacy. You can also search the PharmInfoNet website at www.pharminfo.com and AskAPatient website at www.askapatient.com for consumer ratings on drugs. Package inserts of prescription medications, over-the-counter drugs, and some herbal remedies contain detailed information about directions for use, contraindications, and adverse reactions.

Libraries & Bookstores

Libraries are an invaluable source of health information. Once you complete a database search of titles, you can get the publications from the library or have them sent to you for a fee. If the library does not have the book or article you want, it can arrange to borrow it from another library. Libraries stock medical dictionaries, encyclopedias, and health handbooks and maintain lists of community health resources such as support groups and health programs or services.

Library reference services, particularly medical ones, will usually research topics for you for free or a very small fee. These services will provide you with a bibliography of sources from which you can then pick and choose the publications you want.

Library resources for alternative medicine are more limited. This is likely to change as more funds become available for alternative medicine research and libraries are encouraged to purchase more books on the subject. The widest variety of information on alternative medicine is probably found in retail bookstores and establishments that feature natural health products. Opinions expressed in these publications differ significantly, so be sure to consider and confirm the source of the information before using it.

Do Your Own Research

Government Resources

A wide range of health information on conditions, treatments, and scientific research is available to consumers from state and federal government agencies. Most government agencies also have Internet sites. City and county health agencies can also provide you with information about the health programs that they sponsor or support, which may also be accessible online.

Federal agencies that provide health information to the public include:

Agency for Healthcare Research and Quality
(800) 358–9295 or www.ahrq.gov

Combined Health Information Database (CHID)
chid.nih.gov

Consumer Information
www.consumer.gov

Department of Health and Human Services
(877) 696–6775 or www.hhs.gov
Surgeon General—www.surgeongeneral.gov
National Health Information Center—www.health.gov/nhic
Healthfinder—www.healthfinder.com
National Women's Health Information Center—www.4woman.gov

Federal Information Center (FIC)
(800) 688–9889 or www.fic.info.gov

Food and Drug Administration
(888) 463–6332 or www.fda.gov

Health Information
www.health.gov
www.health.gov/statelocal/

National Institutes of Health (NIH)
www.nih.gov
Institutes & Offices—www.nih.gov/icd/
Phone Numbers—www.nih.gov/news/infoline.htm
Health Information—www.nih.gov/health/

National Center for Complementary and Alternative Medicine (NCCAM)
(888) 644–6226 or nccam.nih.gov

National Library of Medicine
(888) 346–3656 or www.nlm.nih.gov
Med Portal—www.medportal.com
Medline Plus—www.nlm.nih.gov/medlineplus
Pub Med—www.nlm.nih.gov/entrez/query.fcgi

Organ Donations
www.organdonor.gov

Substance Abuse and Mental Health Services
www.samhsa.gov

8

Engage in Health Self-Care

When we hear the term health self-care, we usually think of prevention, but it involves much more than that. Self-care involves an ongoing personal commitment to take an active role in your health. It can be defined as anything you do to effect good health, whether you are trying to get well or you want to stay well.

Health self-care includes everything from engaging in healthy lifestyle habits to taking an herb to alleviate the side effects of a pharmaceutical drug to doing nothing in order to reduce stress or allow an injury to heal. Responsible self-care can eliminate the need for intervention in the first place or encourage the healing process.

All health professionals acknowledge the benefits of developing healthy lifestyle habits such as good nutrition, regular exercise, adequate rest, and the utilization of stress management techniques. When illness occurs, however, conventional medicine tends to take over with pharmacological drugs and invasive treatments, offering very little guidance on how we can participate in our own care. Once the goal of conventional medicine is reached or all interventions are exhausted, people are often left alone to deal with the aftermath of illness and the consequences of treatment.

The tendency of conventional medicine to assume control during illness and depart when treatment is over, coupled with its tendency to use crisis medicine for relatively benign conditions, necessitates that we become more actively engaged in health self-care.

There are many ways to approach health self-care, which includes all aspects of health—physical, emotional, and spiritual. You, along with your provider, must determine the self-care issues that are appropriate for you.

There are also many different ways to address the same self-care task. For example, we all need regular exercise. You must find the exercise that works best for you, so you will be motivated to perform it on a regular basis. Most of us need to manage daily stress. One person may be able to manage stress by listening to stress reduction audiotapes, but another may need to do it by sitting quietly for a period of time. Ten minutes of quiet may be sufficient time for one person to unwind, but thirty minutes or more may be required for another person to accomplish the same goal.

Engage in Health Self-Care

Self-Care to Promote Health

Self-care issues to promote health are typically associated with good nutrition, regular exercise, adequate rest, and the implementation of stress management techniques. In order to promote health, you might reduce your intake of fast food, stop drinking alcohol, drink more water, or consume more health-promoting foods such as garlic to prevent or alleviate colds. You may want to increase the level of exercise you are already performing, cease performing an exercise that may be causing you harm, initiate a holistic exercise such as yoga or *tai chi*, or follow prescribed physical therapy exercises.

Relaxation programs can be initiated or modified in various ways. You can engage in daily stress management through the use of breathing exercises, relaxation tapes, or self-hypnosis. Television viewing time can be reduced, and nightly caffeine avoided in order to enhance better sleep.

Self-care to promote health can involve the regular use of devices such as an "S hook" (a contraption for kneading tight muscles), a dental retainer to straighten teeth, a protective bandage for a soft tissue injury, or a zabuton or special pillow to meditate. Self-care also includes caring for a wound and keeping a diary of the effects of a medicine or treatment.

The development of a good attitude is an important self-care task to promote health. It is especially challenging to do this in the presence of illness or another adversarial situation over which you feel you have little control. Many of us need to simplify our lives by reducing our daily schedules and downsizing our activities. We can also recognize and eliminate self-induced stressors, difficult situations that we create for ourselves unnecessarily and quite often unconsciously.

Sometimes, health self-care is a matter of employing a simple technique or engaging in an activity for a limited period of time. Other times, it is about making major, permanent changes in lifestyle and attitude.

Self-Care & the Environment

Learning to protect yourself from environmental impediments to health is a relatively new self-care issue and is more likely to be addressed by an alternative medicine provider than a conventional one. An estimated 65,000 chemicals are released into our environment by industrialization and technological advancements. As a result of this, environmental illness (EI) is on the rise and has become a serious health concern in our society.

Toxic building materials like asbestos, the proximity of electrical power lines, improperly prepared or stored food, impure drinking water, pesticides, whether they are in the soil of the food you buy at the grocery store or are used to kill household pests, and common cleaning agents are believed to contribute to a variety of health problems including many forms of cancer. Our environment can also be emotionally toxic if it includes people with negative attitudes and behaviors.

Whether your environment is the actual cause of illness or merely makes things worse, common sense dictates that you do as much as possible to eliminate harmful elements from it. As both a prevention and intervention necessity, we must evaluate and make adjustments to our physical environment in order to enhance and maintain our health.

Self-care to Reduce the Effects of Medicine

Along with promoting health, self-care interventions can significantly reduce or ameliorate the adverse effects of conventional medical treatment and drugs. Certain foods can be used to promote healthy intestinal flora that is damaged by antibiotics, reduce nausea from invasive treatments such as chemotherapy, and enhance immunity that is suppressed or compromised by prescription drugs.

Self-care to reduce the effects of medicine frequently involves the use of alternative medicine remedies and herbs, which can also address all of the above. Alternative medicine can also be utilized before and after medical surgery to counteract its effects and to facilitate recovery.

Physical exercises and prescribed movements reduce pain and increase flexibility, balancing the flow of energy throughout the body, which can be disrupted with conventional treatment. Stress management techniques and breathing exercises bring clarity to the mood-altering effects of certain prescription drugs and the disorientation that usually accompanies illness. Conventional treatment and drugs often interfere with sleep, but there are many things you can do on your own to assure rest without taking additional medications.

Self-Care & Alternative Medicine

One of the basic premises behind alternative medicine is that people should be actively involved not only in the maintenance of their health but also in their recovery from illness. Documenting changes in your physical, emotional, and spiritual condition is an important part of this responsibility. Alternative medicine's success is entirely dependent on your willingness to assume this role and address these issues, and providers encourage a high level of participation to ensure a positive outcome from alternative treatment.

Self-care in alternative medicine can mean many things, depending on the alternative practice. In Chinese medicine, self-care includes cooking and drinking a raw herb tea mixture, taking Chinese patent medicines several times a day, engaging in disciplines such as *tai chi* or *qigong*, receiving massage, and performing special breathing exercises.

Self-care in the use of homeopathy involves avoiding antidotal substances such as coffee and camphor. In ayurvedic medicine, self-care involves following a particular diet, practicing yoga, taking an herbal formula, using aromatherapy, engaging in meditation, and performing dry brush massage.

Unfortunately, health self-care is still not taken very seriously in our culture. We are aware of the importance of engaging in healthy lifestyle habits, but most of us do not take action until disaster strikes. We wait until we are faced with our mortality or the mortality of someone we love in order to take action.

Engage in Health Self-Care

To engage in health self-care requires focus, effort, discipline, and resolve, but there are more resources for health self-care available to consumers than ever before. You do not have to feel helpless in the face of any health crisis. Understanding that you can have a direct impact on your health through the adoption of certain practices, lifestyle changes, and interventions is an empowering realization and a critical step toward recovery.

☑ Check List

1. Health self-care is anything you do to effect good health—whether it is used to maintain health or to recover from illness or injury.

2. Self-care is helpful in reducing the harmful effects of conventional medicine and is integral in the use of alternative medicine.

3. The most common self-care issues involve diet, exercise, stress, rest, and the environment.

4. You and your health care provider must determine the self-care issues that are appropriate for you.

5. Once you decide on a self-care issue, you must find the approach to it that works best for you.

6. One of the keys to successful self-care is regular application and practice.

9

Connect with Medical Support Staff

Communication is the cornerstone of any health care relationship. It can sometimes be enhanced when you form a positive and productive alliance with someone other than the health care provider. The basis for good communication with a provider often begins with a member of his staff who serves as a link between you and the provider. This person may be the only connection you have to the provider, particularly in busy medical offices, and in most cases, it will be a registered nurse, family nurse practitioner, or physician assistant.

We all know that conventional medical offices and clinics, particularly multipractice ones that are located in large cities, are usually hierarchical and often chaotic. Big medical establishments are also notorious for inadequate communication with their clients.

In these environments, it is not uncommon for providers to intentionally limit their accessibility, although this is an odd priority for any health professional who is truly committed to the welfare of his clientele. Some providers simply refuse to interact with clients outside of the appointment time.

Medical schools and training programs frequently fail to emphasize the importance of good communication and positive, collaborative partnerships with consumers to the extent that they should. Since providers have many patients and concerns other than your welfare and you have only one doctor, the burden falls upon you to ensure good communication with a provider any way you can. It is simply unrealistic to think that it could be any other way.

Family Nurse Practitioners & Physician Assistants

Registered nurses have been around a long time, but family nurse practitioners and physician assistants are relatively new to the health care industry. More and more medical doctors employ nurse practitioners and physician assistants to alleviate the increasing burden upon them because these professionals can perform many of the same functions.

Although nurse practitioners and physician assistants have similar roles, they have different origins and their training is founded on different educational models and theoretical bases. They also operate under different state laws.

Family nurse practitioners (FNP or NP) are typically educated as advanced practice nurses at the master or post-master degree levels and are licensed by the state. There are also nurse practitioner training programs that are merely the equivalent of a two-year junior college.

Nurse practitioners perform histories and examinations, order and interpret diagnostic tests, treat acute and manage chronic illnesses, provide counseling for healthy lifestyle habits and self-care skills, and prescribe medication. Nurse practitioners work either collaboratively with the medical doctor or completely on their own. They can be found in a variety of health care settings, including medical offices, clinics, hospitals, and chronic care facilities.

Physician assistants (PA) come from a variety of health backgrounds and are typically educated at the bachelor or master degree levels. Some physician assistant training programs do not offer a degree but only a certificate. Medical school-based programs have developed over the past two decades to meet an increasing demand for physician assistants.

Unlike nurse practitioners, physician assistants are not licensed and must always work under the supervision of a medical doctor. They also do not have the medical training of nurses and earn less money than nurses or nurse practitioners. Physician assistants can also be found in medical offices, clinics, and hospital settings, where they sometimes assist doctors during medical surgery.

Advantages

There are many benefits to developing a relationship with a nurse or other support staff:

- *accessibility*—you can reach them more easily on the phone.
- *time*—they have more of it to answer your questions.
- *information*—they can relay it to you in terms you can understand.
- *support*—they are better hand-holders.

It is usually easier to talk to a nurse than a doctor. Nurses understand the complications from treatment and can help you reduce the possibility of their occurrence. They can assist you with self-care issues by explaining what you can do on your own to facilitate treatment. Nurses can also handle the more mundane aspects of treatment, such as providing you with copies of medical records and diagnostic reports.

The biggest advantage to developing a relationship with a nurse or other medical support staff is better access to and communication with the health care provider. Their role is to serve you as well as assist their employers, so it makes sense for you to utilize their skills as much as possible.

Disadvantages

You do not want to develop a relationship with a nurse or other medical staff member to the extent that it becomes a substitute or replacement for your relationship with the provider. Some providers encourage their support staff to perform an expanded role by routinely having them field calls from clients to answer their questions. For simple matters such as prescription refills, this is acceptable. For serious concerns about treatment and outcome, it is not. To avoid this situation, make it clear to support staff when you want to speak directly to the provider.

Not everyone who works in a medical office wants to assume a supportive role or is encouraged to do so. Some medical staff behave as though their most important task is to keep you *from* the doctor instead of facilitating access *to* him. These people take themselves and their positions much too seriously. Try to avoid negative medical personnel at all costs because of the detrimental effect it can have on the entire health care experience.

By virtue of their training, nurses and their counterparts do not possess the medical knowledge of providers, even though they sometimes have a comparable amount of practical experience. Information that they offer you about your medical care and treatment should always be confirmed with the provider.

The accessibility of nurses is decreasing because their ranks have been significantly reduced in recent years. Nurses are leaving the profession in record numbers due to retirement, inadequate compensation, and unsatisfactory working conditions. They point to understaffing, excessive stress, and the physical demands of jobs as the causes of poor working conditions. This labor shortage is reaching critical proportions and has contributed to escalating hospitals costs. Recent surveys predict a nationwide shortage of nurses in the very near future.

Alternative Medicine

Alternative medicine providers typically do not employ registered nurses, family nurse practitioners, or physician assistants, unless the provider is also a medical doctor. Alternative providers usually work alone, but if they employ anyone, it is typically a secretary or receptionist.

There are definite advantages to the consumer in this situation. Alternative providers are more accessible and will call you back personally because there is usually no one else to do it. Although there is less of an opportunity to develop a relationship with someone other than the alternative provider, there is also less of a need for it. As alternative medicine becomes more conventional, this will probably change.

Unsung Heroes

Registered nurses and their contemporary counterparts belong to probably the most undervalued profession in health care. They comprise the backbone of conventional medicine and fill an emotional and psychological void that is created and perpetuated by a bureaucratic health care system. In fact, without nurses, nurse practitioners, and physician assistants, the flaws and inadequacies of our system of medicine would be much more obvious to us than they already are. Without them, the health care profession would be in a very sorry state.

Nurses have always served as powerful advocates for consumers, even though they receive scant credit for doing so. They possess the training, education, skill, knowledge, and hands-on experience to be effective health educators and promoters, critical roles often overlooked by the system they serve. Nurses sometimes possess nearly as much practical knowledge about and experience with medical conditions and treatments as providers.

Connect with Medical Support Staff

An experienced nurse, nurse practitioner, or physician assistant can be your best ally in a health care crisis. Their value becomes even more evident in a hospital setting where they often assume the mantle of coordinating your care and compensating for a sterile, impersonal hospital environment.

Nurses and their contemporary counterparts provide physical and emotional care in contrast to the provider's technological skill. These important health advocates are ever present and accomplished at listening, supporting, assisting, understanding, informing, and resolving important health issues as they arise.

10

Network with Other Consumers

Consumers are powerful allies to one another in health care, particularly in the use of alternative medicine. Knowing what you want from health care and having the ability to communicate it as effectively and assertively as possible are critical in any health care relationship. Connecting with other consumers will help you to do this.

Connections with health care consumers provide you with two important resources—support and information. Support or information provided by consumers differs from that provided by health professionals in point of view and experience. As such, consumers are an invaluable resource for making informed health care choices.

The best sources of support and information are from people you know and trust. You can also connect with health consumers on the Internet, in support groups, community health agencies, and hospital outpatient programs. The Internet has chat rooms, discussion groups, and "mailing lists" such as CataList and Liszt, allowing you to connect with people from all over the world. You can also meet health consumers at health fairs, workshops, seminars, and natural food or other health-oriented retail establishments. There are numerous books and articles written by consumers who possess firsthand experience with medical treatment.

As with any health resource, always consider the source of the information and verify it with reliable, independent parties.

Information

Health consumers can generally point you in the right direction, narrowing your choices and reducing costly trial and error. Proactive consumers will swap objective, uncensored information with you about the latest medical studies and treatments and the best providers and medical facilities. They will tell you what no one else will.

Consumers can steer you away from bad providers, although you should keep in mind that what is bad to one person may not be bad to another. Those in the know can also guide you to the best resources, saving you the time and expense of sorting through voluminous amounts of information on your own.

Consumer collaborations are especially helpful in the use of alternative medicine, which is still very much a word-of-mouth business. Alternative medicine choices can seem endless to the person who is ill or the inexperienced user. Shopping around for alternative treatments is expensive, and information on alternative medicine can be confusing. The alternative practice may not be regulated or eligible for insurance benefits, and there may be very little, if any, scientific data on its effectiveness. Some people may simply want to use alternative medicine on their own.

Learning about alternative medicine from others is only helpful to a certain point because it is highly individualized and its effectiveness depends on a variety of factors. Just because it works for one person does not mean that it will work for you.

Support

Consumers today are challenged by the task of developing and maintaining meaningful relationships with others in the presence of technological developments that seem to distance us further and further from one another. We are also extremely mobile. Technology detaches us from personal human contact, and mobility causes relationships to be temporary and short-term—big hurdles to overcome in the midst of a health crisis.

Emotional connections are an important component of maintaining and improving your health. Not only is this logical, but it has also been documented in many scientific studies. Research has linked greater immunity with social supports, and positive outcomes were also demonstrated from participation in support groups for coronary heart disease and breast cancer.

Support groups kill two birds with one stone. They provide consumers not only with emotional support but also an environment for the dissemination of practical information. Support groups with a particular focus, such as cancer or arthritis, offer participants information that is specific to their condition along with the comfort that comes from being in the company of people who can truly identify with each other's experiences.

Of course, the best sources of encouragement in a health crisis are from family and friends. Unfortunately, not everyone is blessed with this type of emotional support. In times of illness, many people are forced to make new connections and create a support system during a health crisis. Others turn to their faith and seek fellowship through members of a religious or spiritual community.

Your health care provider can also be a source of emotional support. But the support you receive from a health professional differs in perspective from the support offered by another health care consumer, particularly if the former happens to be part of the problem for which you need the emotional support.

Your local library, hospital, county social service department, and telephone directory have listings of support services in your community. Many support services do not advertise, so it is wise to ask around about services that are available in your area.

Almost every organization with a health focus, such as the Cancer Society, Arthritis Foundation, Diabetes Society, and Kidney Foundation, has information on support services. The Center for Attitudinal Healing, based in California but with centers nationwide, offers free group support for a variety of physical and emotional conditions.

11

Request Copies of Records & Reports

Consumer access to medical records and diagnostic reports is necessary in becoming more involved in your health care. This data helps you to prepare for health care appointments, which was discussed in Chapter 5, and contributes to your health literacy.

Health literacy has been shown in research studies to affect health outcome. Consumers with poor health literacy reported worse health status, less understanding of medical conditions, and were more likely to be hospitalized. We can conclude from this that increased health literacy results in better health outcomes. Learning to understand your treatment records and reports is one way to accomplish this.

There are many health care providers who will argue that you do not possess the training or expertise to understand your medical records and diagnostic reports. They may warn you that your attempts to do so will lead to misinterpretation, overreaction, and potential disaster.

There is no question that the terminology contained in medical records is complex, and everyone knows it is impossible to read a doctor's handwriting. But you will never be able to understand your records until you have access to them and your doctor takes the time to explain them to you. This should be a non-negotiable part of the health care relationship, an investment in your education every provider should be willing to make.

Access to Medical Records

Access to federal medical records is protected by federal law. Under the Freedom of Information Act of 1966 and the Federal Privacy Act of 1974, people have a right to their medical records. The Freedom of Information Clearinghouse provides assistance to people in getting their medical records.

The Consumer Information Center at P.O. Box 100, Pueblo, Colorado, 81002 provides a free booklet to consumers titled *Your Right to Federal Records*. For a small fee, the Public Citizen Health Research Group at (202) 833–3000 provides a booklet to consumers titled *Medical Records: Getting Yours*.

In most instances, access to medical records is protected by state law. If your right to medical records is not protected by state law, it is a medical right upon which you should still insist. There are few exceptions to this rule. Providers may be exempt from giving you access to your records if they can show that doing so would be injurious to your health in some manner.

Most providers will give you access and a copy of your medical records upon request. If you can better understand your condition and treatment through these records, providers can better do their job. They also want to keep your business.

It was previously noted that providers can authorize you to receive copies of diagnostic test results. They can do this merely by adding "copy patient" on the test orders. Some laboratories will also provide you with copies of test results upon request, and you can also sign for and receive your original x-ray films. You pay for medical tests through premiums, deductibles, copayments, or payment in full, so you should have no qualms about insisting on receiving copies of these reports.

Utilize Records & Reports

Take copies of your medical records and diagnostic reports with you to health care appointments, so providers can help you understand them. These documents expedite treatment with a new provider, especially in the presence of a serious health condition. When you know what treatments and tests have and have not been performed, you can also avoid the unnecessary duplication and error that regularly occur in health care.

Although access to medical records in and of itself does not guarantee good treatment, it allows you to be more active in the health care process, which makes good treatment more likely.

Records that you bring to a medical office are your property and must be returned to you upon request. If medical records are sent to a medical office by another provider, you may be charged a fee for photocopies.

If you travel for work or move frequently, having your medical records with you can be an advantage. You also have the option of discontinuing a relationship with a provider without having to contact him again. In the event of a medical emergency, having a copy of your medical records may even save your life.

Medical Information Board (MIB)

The Medical Information Board (MIB) maintains a database of insurance underwriting information. A report by the MIB is created if you have made an application for life, health, or disability insurance in the past seven years or if an insurance underwriting investigation revealed a condition that could affect your health or longevity. Information contained in the report may be accessed by health insurers if you apply for coverage and can affect your application approval and premiums.

Every person should secure a report from the Medical Information Board (MIB). Contact the MIB at P.O. Box 105, Essex Station, Boston, Massachusetts, 02112, telephone (617) 426–3660, and ask for a Request for Disclosure (Form D–2). You can also access this document online at www.mib.com.

Request Copies of Records & Reports

Take the Time

Take the time to maintain a copy of your medical records and diagnostic reports and learn to understand them. This will help you to complete another important task, tracking your progress from medical treatment, which is discussed in the following chapter.

The ability to read and understand your medical records takes time, like learning any new language, but it is no longer feasible to leave this task solely to providers. The common thread in all of the steps outlined in this guide is to assume a more active role in health care. As a responsible consumer, you cannot allow any persons, particularly those with multiple priorities, to be in charge of your care.

In conventional medicine, medical records and diagnostic tests determine the course of treatment. When you understand your condition, at least as defined by these documents, you can contribute to its resolution by making informed decisions about your care. Contributing to your care also gives you more control over it.

Maintaining a copy of your medical records and diagnostic reports is an important step toward becoming more fully involved in the health care process. Once you have access to this information, you can participate in your care in a way you were never able to before.

12

Track Your Own Progress

If you want to get the most from your health care, you must be willing to monitor change in your condition by tracking your own progress during medical treatment. Monitoring change in your condition is about paying attention to what your body, mind, and spirit tell you that is different from what they were telling you before you received the treatment and about documenting these changes in your condition as accurately as possible. These efforts can result in more efficient, less-costly health care and quicker resolution to health problems. Tracking your own progress is an easy yet empowering task.

The primary methods by which conventional providers monitor change in health conditions are provider observation and diagnostic tests. Although client self-report is taken into account in health decisions, it is clearly marginalized in conventional medicine and takes a back seat to the opinions of doctors and the results of technology. Provider observation and diagnostic tests, however, are not always reliable or accurate. For this reason, greater value should be placed on your opinion and beliefs during the treatment process.

Although conventional medicine does not rely primarily on self-report, alternative medicine does. In alternative medicine, your observations and experiences are highly valued. You are encouraged to note or record your observations and experiences following treatment, so you can accurately relay them to your alternative provider. Health status in alternative medicine is also documented by provider observation, but diagnostic tests are usually only employed as a last resort.

Record Your Observations

When you keep track of your progress during medical treatment, you will note changes in your condition and can record these observations in a daily or weekly journal or diary. These observations can include:

- what you consume
- your level of physical activity
- how well you sleep
- what you dream about
- your emotional states

- changes in disease symptoms
- acute and chronic reactions to treatment, drugs, and herbs

Write your observations down when they occur, so you do not forget them. How you do this is really up to you. Some people carry journals with them and take notes as they go. Others reserve a special time such as bedtime to record their experiences of the day. You can write your observations anywhere—in a journal, health diary, notepad, notebook, or professional organizer.

The method you choose to record your observances is not as important as your consistency in doing it and what it accomplishes for you. Schedule a regular time or day to make these notations, and keep this record in the same place, so you will always know where it is.

Benefits

When you keep track of your progress during medical treatment, you provide yourself and your doctor with critical information about the effects of the treatment. Informed decisions can then be made about the next course of action. Engaging in this simple ritual also reduces the chaos and confusion that frequently surround illness.

People who are willing to monitor their own progress find themselves more aware of their needs and more self-reliant in the health care process. This task not only ensures that you will make the right decisions about your care, but it also increases self-awareness and builds confidence, important qualities for getting and staying well.

Tracking your progress following medical treatment is also a means by which you can prepare for health care appointments, allowing for more efficient use of the appointment time, which is discussed in Chapter 5. Recording your observations about the effects of treatment is also a self-care activity, which is considered in Chapter 8.

Your perception of yourself and your health condition is as important as any provider's observation or diagnostic test, if not more. With practice, you can learn to make connections between health cause and effect and can turn this information into action, making a significant contribution to the healing process. This will ultimately allow you to be alert to a health imbalance long before it becomes a more serious problem.

13

Exercise Patience with Results

You must exercise patience during treatment if you expect to use medicine with any degree of success. This is probably the second most difficult task to master in becoming a better health care consumer, next to asserting yourself with providers.

In our society, we expect frequent medical intervention in the form of a pharmaceutical drug, treatment, or surgery and immediate results to alleviate our pain and suffering and facilitate our recovery from illness. We want our health problems over quickly, and consequently, we tend to ignore or bury the ones that are not easily resolved if we can get away with it. Health problems that are ignored or buried always become much bigger health problems down the road.

We must get over this desire for constant intervention and immediate results in health care. The former is not always necessary, and the latter is not always possible. The need for immediate results in conventional medicine has led to its misuse and abuse. We misuse medicine when we use technology unnecessarily to prolong life and when we use invasive treatments for benign conditions, for which alternative treatments are more appropriate. We abuse medicine when we overtreat people, compromising the body's natural ability to defend itself and causing problems that were not present in the first place.

Constant intervention until it leads to measurable relief comes at a heavy price. In conventional medicine, it results in temporary cures with often permanent physical consequences due to the invasiveness of conventional treatment.

It takes a long time for the body to get into a state of imbalance in which illness is manifested. It would then follow that it takes a commensurate amount of time to get the body back into a state of balance and harmony. Allowing an intervention to work properly or the natural ability of the body to right itself on its own is essential for the person who truly wants lasting results.

Alternative Medicine

In alternative medicine, there is simply no such thing as a short-term cure. Although a sudden improvement in your condition can sometimes happen, it usually takes longer to achieve results because of the way the medicine is designed to work. It can take weeks, months, or even years to resolve

Exercise Patience with Results

a health imbalance, requiring different alternative interventions for different stages of healing.

Sometimes, you need to make dramatic changes in lifestyle to facilitate healing, which takes time. Symptoms can also become worse before getting better, which tests your patience even more than merely waiting for results.

In noncrisis conditions, for which the use of alternative medicine is preferable, there is no need for immediate results and improvement in your condition can be achieved without constant intervention. Sometimes, the proper course of action in alternative medicine is no intervention at all, allowing a previous treatment to work or giving the body a chance to regain a sense of balance on its own. Constant intervention in alternative medicine can also have a negative impact on treatment and create the potential for harm.

Although most people still want to take a pill and defer health decisions to others, those who use alternative medicine on a regular basis learn that there is no quick fix or magic bullet that leads to true healing. True healing, which can be stimulated or encouraged from the outside, arises from within.

People who expect instant, lasting results from an herbal remedy or an alternative treatment are going to be sorely disappointed. The effective use of alternative medicine requires a self-reliance quite different from the self-reliance that is expected of us in the use of conventional medicine.

Changing Perceptions & Expectations

Exercising patience with the results of medical intervention requires a major shift in attitude. In order to do this, we must change our perception of health care from an enterprise that solves our problems to one that enhances our own ability to solve our problems. We can also change our overall expectation of health care from immediate and temporary results to time-consuming and long-lasting resolution.

Being assertive with health care providers requires an understanding that you have the right to participate fully in the process of your own care. Being patient with medical results requires an understanding that there is no quick fix with the use of any medicine and that immediate results can have negative consequences.

In order to change your perception and expectation of health care, you must change both your attitude and behavior toward it. Cognitive experts believe that if you change your attitude first, your behavior will change. Behavioral experts believe that if you change your behavior first, a change in attitude will automatically follow. The former means that if you understand the importance of being patient, you will behave patiently. The latter means that if you behave patiently for a long enough period of time, you will eventually comprehend the importance of it.

These two approaches are often characterized by psychotherapists as "from the head down" or "from the heart up." You must determine the method of change that works best for you.

We expect immediate gratification and constant intervention in many aspects of our lives. Changing your perceptions and expectations of health care can have a positive impact on your life. If you can learn to exercise patience

Exercise Patience with Results

with health care results, you can also wait for what truly fulfills and satisfies you in life.

An integral part of the growth and healing process is to be at some degree of peace with yourself in the face of adversity. If you can change your expectations of health care, you will clearly maximize its benefits.

14

Know Your Health Care Rights

Americans take their legal rights very seriously. In fact, we may have more practicing lawyers per square inch than the Gobi Desert has sand. The whole concept of health care rights is an ironic one since there really should be no priority in health care other than your health. It is a relatively new concept, having arisen out of the gatekeeper mentality and profit-making sensibility that has overtaken our health care system.

As we have already considered, there are many priorities in health care other than your health. In some ways, health care rights are a necessary evil that we must now define in order to protect ourselves from the escalating autocracy of medicine.

Is Your Health Care Killing You?

The legislation of health care rights began in earnest with the Federal Public Health Act of 1947, and there have been many modifications and additions to health care law during the past fifty years. In the new century, health care rights are in a state of great flux and crisis. Many health care rights are protected by state law, while others are protected by federal law.

Federal law on health care rights includes the following:

- Family and Medical Leave Act of 1993 provides job protection in circumstances of illness or pregnancy.

- Americans with Disabilities Act of 1990 grants protections to people with disabilities.

- Health Insurance Portability and Accountability Act of 1996 ensures continued insurance coverage for people who lose or change their jobs.

- Child Health Insurance Program of 1997 assists low-income families.

A National Treatment Plan Initiative, recently introduced by the federal government, requires insurance companies to provide benefits for mental illness and drug addiction on a parity with other illnesses. A Patient Bill of Rights, introduced by the government in 1999 but yet to pass both houses of Congress, is directed at HMOs. This bill allows consumers to hold health plans accountable for their actions but will do little to improve outcomes or the quality of health care that is received.

Know Your Health Care Rights

Although health care advocates agree that consumers should have an inherent right to self-determination—free choice of action without external compulsion—this is a right that managed care has effectively tried to limit or do away with altogether.

Another hotly debated health care right involves the confidentiality of medical records. This has become an important legal issue, arising from abuses by insurance companies in their efforts to get more information than they need to process claims and from the inevitability of electronic medical records, which will make confidential medical records accessible by computer. One suggestion to address this problem is to allow doctors to submit summaries of treatment to regulators, so you do not have to censor what you tell your doctor for fear it will be used against you to deny benefits or increase your premiums.

The Clinton administration issued the first comprehensive standards to protect the privacy of medical records. These standards required providers to obtain written consent from consumers before disclosing any medical information and to limit the disclosure of personal health information by hard or electronic copy. Unfortunately, these standards were recently modified by the Bush administration due to resistance from both health providers and insurance companies.

The Joint Commission on Accreditation of Healthcare Organizations (JCAHO), which oversees almost 5,000 hospitals nationwide, recently approved a package of patient safety standards in an effort to reduce the occurrence of medical mistakes. This action was taken as a result of the explosive report referred to earlier that almost 100,000 hospital patients die annually as a result of preventable errors. Medical mistakes also cost hospitals up to $29 billion in lost wages, disability payments, and additional medical care.

The new safety standards imposed by the JCAHO include a requirement that hospitals tell the truth to patients when mistakes are made instead of trying to cover them up in order to avoid legal liability. Failure to comply with these new standards can result in loss of accreditation. Hospitals that belong to the American Hospital Association (AHA) also adhere to a 1973 Bill of Rights, which protects hospitalized consumers.

In the absence of comprehensive federal law on health care, many state legislatures have introduced or passed their own initiatives on issues such as access to medical services and confidentiality of medical records. According to the National Conference of State Legislatures, health care issues made up the largest proportion of bills introduced in state legislatures in 1999.

Many states have their own Patient Bill of Rights. *Any willing provider* laws exist in 21 states, which require insurance companies to accept out-of-network providers at the insurer's rate and contract terms. It may be interesting to note that Kentucky's any willing provider law was recently upheld by the U.S. Supreme Court.

Every state has *mandatory benefit laws*, requiring insurers to provide benefits for designated services. Some of the services are unusual, such as sex change operations, but many of them are routine, such as mammograms. An insurance company must pay for these services even if they are listed as excluded benefits in your health plan.

Please note that insurers are not obligated to disclose state mandatory benefit laws to subscribers. However, the

National Association of Insurance Commissioners maintains a website at www.naic.org where you can research state benefit laws and cross-reference them with your insurance policy for discrepancies.

Top 20 Health Care Rights

Health care rights cannot protect you unless you exercise them, and you cannot exercise them unless you know what they are. Whether or not they are protected by state or federal law, you can still insist on exercising a right that you believe is important to your health and well-being. Responsible providers will comply with any reasonable request if they value your business.

The *Top 20 Health Care Rights* are:

1. You have a right to review your medical records.
2. You have a right to receive copies of test results.
3. You have a right to know if a doctor has a financial interest in a health care organization to which you may be referred.
4. You have a right to know if a doctor was professionally disciplined by a medical licensing board.
5. You have a right to question an insurance company's denial of coverage with the insurer and the state agency that regulates insurance companies.
6. You have a right to have someone present with you in the examining room.

7. You have the right to refuse medical intervention to prolong your life.

8. You have a right to be fully informed about your medical condition. Doctors can refuse to disclose information only if they can demonstrate that doing so would be detrimental to your health.

9. You have a right to emergency care from a hospital regardless of your ability to pay if not having it would cause your condition to worsen. Once you have been admitted to a hospital, you cannot be discharged because you cannot pay.

10. You have the right to know if you are participating in a medical experiment.

11. You have a right to medical privacy and patient-provider confidentiality unless you sue a doctor or other provider.

12. You have a right to informed consent, which means that a doctor cannot subject you to any treatment without your permission. A doctor must also disclose all treatment options and alternatives, including experimental treatment, even if you cannot afford it.

13. You have a right to know all the risks associated with a medical treatment and to refuse any medical treatment.

14. You have a right to leave a hospital without the consent of the doctor, appeal the discharge notice from a hospital, or transfer to another hospital.

15. You have a right to receive an acceptable level of medical care known as the "The Standard of Practice Doctrine." When treatment falls below the standard of practice dictated by state licensing boards, medical malpractice occurs.

16. You can refuse to be examined by medical students or interns, commonly found in teaching clinics and hospitals.

17. You have a right to a second opinion.

18. You have a right to designate an advocate to make health care decisions for you in the event of incapacitation, withhold life-sustaining procedures in the event of terminal illness, and refuse to resuscitate in the event of cardiac or respiratory arrest.

19. You have a right to health insurance if you lose or quit your job.

20. You have a right to job protection if you become ill or pregnant.

Insurance Companies

Insisting on a health care right with an insurance company can be nothing less than a David and Goliath experience. Health insurer horror stories are plentiful, enough to fill several books. Problems often begin before you ever file a claim. For example, one subscriber received three conflicting interpretations of a policy benefit from three different claims representatives before the service was ever received. When benefits for the service were denied and the subscriber complained about the misinformation, the insurer said in its refusal to reverse its decision that it was the subscriber's responsibility to know the correct interpretation of the benefit!

Another subscriber was misled about the role of underwriting in a transfer application during an application process for initial membership. Two years later, the insurer, a major California carrier, increased the family's premiums to 360% of the original rate in approving their transfer to another plan, recategorizing them from the lowest to the highest risk based on exactly the same medical history.

If you become seriously ill, the time when your rights are most likely to be at risk, many insurance companies would love to have you cancel your policy with them and go elsewhere. They often cease being your friend and can even become adversarial when the benefits that they pay to you exceed the premiums that you pay to them.

You must pay your insurance premiums on time because insurers can and do cancel policies for late payment, especially if you are ill and costing them money. Insurance companies also make mistakes when they process claims, so you should always review your explanation of benefits for possible errors because errors can cost you higher premiums.

If an insurer unfairly denies you coverage for a health benefit (i.e., in violation of your policy or the state mandatory benefit laws) and the appeals process with the insurer has been completely exhausted, you have recourse with whatever government agency regulates insurance companies in your state. This agency will usually be the Department of Insurance, Department of Consumer Affairs, or state Attorney General (see Appendix A).

State agencies that monitor and regulate insurance companies have a grievance process by which you can submit a complaint about a health insurer to a claims services bureau. Your complaint will be investigated for violations of state law and judged by a presumably competent and impartial claims officer.

State regulatory agencies can be useful in resolving unnecessary delays in the processing of claims and unfair denial of benefits, but some agencies function more effectively than others. Despite what you may think or have been led to believe, you *can* exercise some control over an insurer.

Unless an employer is paying part or all of your health insurance, the Health Insurance Portability and Accountability Act of 1996 allows individuals to shop around for insurance without the penalties that were typically imposed in the past. This federal law is designed to protect people who lose or change their jobs from losing their health insurance and applies to both group and individual coverage. It means that you cannot be denied coverage if, for any reason, your insurance ends or is canceled. Insurance companies can still discriminate against new subscribers by setting the amount of the premiums as high or as low as they want based on your previous medical history.

If you have private or employer-provided health insurance, you should familiarize yourself with the maximum lifetime benefit your insurance company will pay for your care, the treatments and services that are covered by your policy, and coverage for pre-existing exclusions. If you are older, you should determine your eligibility for Medicare or Medicaid and the benefit limitations of these programs.

It is important that you read the full certificate of coverage of your insurance policy rather than a summary of coverage because critical information is omitted from the summary. If the full certificate of coverage is not provided to you, request a copy of it.

Insurance for alternative medicine is extremely limited and usually only covers those services provided or authorized by a medical doctor, osteopath, or chiropractor. To make matters worse, many medical doctors who practice alternative medicine are opting to discontinue participation in health plans because of the difficulties involved in getting paid for their services.

An advantage to using alternative medicine is the fact that insurance companies are usually not involved, and you have more control over your care without having to deal with annoying, third-party involvement. The main disadvantage to using alternative medicine, of course, is that you must assume all of the costs yourself.

Legal Complaints

If your legal rights have been violated by any health care entity and you have been unable to resolve your complaint through all the normal bureaucratic channels, you may want to consult with a plaintiff's attorney who specializes in such claims. Insurance companies, whether they are acting on behalf of doctors or themselves, will also hire attorneys to represent them in legal complaints. However, you enter into another arena when you legally go after a health provider or health insurer. There are some basic facts you should know before becoming involved in litigation.

Most reputable attorneys will not take your case in the first place unless you are seriously injured and your case is potentially worth at least $100,000 because of the costs associated with litigation. If you are suing a medical doctor, you must find another medical doctor to testify that what the former did to you was below the standard of care for the health care practice. This is not as easy as it seems.

Most doctors are unwilling to testify in medical malpractice claims and will refuse to even treat you if you intend to pursue such a claim. In many instances, you do not know that a doctor has acted incompetently or negligently unless another doctor tells you so. New doctors can and do withhold such information if they believe it will result in a legal complaint against a colleague. Those doctors who are willing to testify against other doctors in malpractice claims will sometimes only do so if the doctor being sued is located out of state. The bottom line is that doctors go to enormous lengths to protect other doctors, regardless of what they have done to harm you.

Once you make it over this hurdle, you must then deal with the insurer. Insurance companies, whether they are representing providers or are being sued directly, are notorious for their unwillingness to fairly or expeditiously settle legitimate claims, dragging the legal process out for years until you tire of it or run out of money to pursue your claim. Attorneys who are hired by insurance companies are typically paid on an hourly basis, so there is little or no incentive for them to resolve your case quickly. Only if your policy or contract with a health insurer requires the use of mandatory binding arbitration or if the insurer is unusually cooperative are legal claims resolved in a reasonable amount of time.

Quick and cost-effective dispute resolution should be available to all consumers with legal claims valued at less than $100,000. The legal process for larger claims should be expedited, and runaway jury awards should be rectified through the appeal's process, which is already in place to deal with such occurrences.

If the agencies with authority over insurers and providers did a better job of disciplining them, there would be less of a need to seek justice through legal action. If you do decide to pursue this course of action, be prepared for a lengthy and arduous legal process.

Although we live in an overly litigious world, we also live in a world in which people are frequently hurt by preventable medical and regulatory errors. We seem to have lost the ability to resolve our own differences in an amicable or mutually satisfactory manner, which is evidenced by the number of court shows on television. Consumers are certainly responsible for frivolous legal claims and have difficulty distinguishing between true harm and a bad result that is no one's fault. But health professionals also make avoidable mistakes, sometimes serious ones, and should be held accountable for their actions.

If you believe that any health care entity has violated your legal rights, make sure that your claim has merit, and do everything possible to encourage its fair resolution *before* you initiate legal action.

Tax Returns

If you file a tax return with either the federal government or state in which you reside, certain medical expenses are deductible from your income. If you pay medical expenses for someone other than yourself, you may have certain tax exemptions on your return, such as claiming the person as a dependent. Paying someone's medical expenses may also qualify as a tax-free gift. Consult with a certified public accountant, tax specialist, or federal and state tax board to determine the tax rights to which you are entitled.

Advance Health Care Directive

Your health care rights include the assurance that your wishes are carried out regarding your care and treatment. The legal document that outlines these rights is called an advance health care directive, and every adult should have one.

An advance health care directive details your wishes for prolonging or sustaining your life with medical intervention and for resuscitation from cardiac or respiratory arrest, known as a *Do Not Resuscitate* (DNR) order. Advance health care directives are not only for people who are seriously ill but also for those who want to be prepared for a medical emergency.

An advance health care directive can designate a health care advocate, someone who makes decisions on your behalf in the event of physical or emotional incapacitation. Designating a health care advocate ensures that your wishes, as outlined in the advance health care directive, are not misinterpreted or ignored by medical personnel.

Advance health care directives are usually part of a living will, living trust, or health care power of attorney, also termed a *durable power of attorney for health care*. You can have an attorney create this document for you, or you can create one yourself. Most books on health care rights cite examples of advance health care directives.

If you create your own advance health care directive, it must conform to state law in order to ensure that it will be upheld by the courts. Consult the law in your state for specific requirements. The directive should also be clearly written to avoid misinterpretation. Advance health care directives should always be witnessed and notarized.

Information on Health Care Rights

Information on state-mandated health care rights is available from your representatives in the state legislature. Information on federally mandated health care rights is available from your U.S. Congressional representatives. The U.S. Department of Health and Human Services also makes information available to consumers on federal health care rights.

State agencies such as the Department of Consumer Affairs, Department of Health and Human Services, and Department of Insurance can provide you with information on state health care rights. State Departments of Mental Health can advise you on mental health rights. County and law school libraries have books that document both federal and state health law, including the original Public Health Act of 1947.

State medical licensing boards set standards of care for health care providers and the basis for professional disciplinary action. These standards apply to any provider who is licensed by the state, including providers of alternative medicine practices such as acupuncture, naturopathy, and massage. Disciplinary actions can take the form of a reprimand or a suspension or revocation of the license to practice. If you receive treatment from a state-licensed provider, you have greater recourse if something goes wrong than you do with an unlicensed one.

Professional associations for conventional and alternative providers also set standards to which members must adhere in order to retain their membership. Information about sanctions against members of professional associations may or may not be available to the public.

There are many publications on health care rights. To adequately address this issue requires an entire book and one that is current, since rights are constantly being revised and modified. Many books on health care rights not only describe what your rights are but also provide comprehensive lists of whom to contact about them, including state agencies, licensing boards, and professional associations.

The American Civil Liberties Union (ACLU) regularly publishes books on health care rights. There are also books about your rights as they specifically relate to insurance companies such as *Making Them Pay: How to Get the Most from Health Insurance and Managed Care* (2001) by attorney Rhonda Orin.

Consumer Advocacy Groups & Health Rights Organizations

There are organizations that deal exclusively with health care rights and others that assist health care consumers, monitor the health care industry, and promote consumer choice (see Appendix B).

Beware of the word "advocate" in the titles of health care organizations. There are hospitals, providers, and insurance companies that use this word or variations of it to promote the sale of their services and products. In these instances, they are only advocates for themselves.

☑ Check List

1. Familiarize yourself with your federal and state health care rights.

2. Know the terms and conditions of your health insurance policy, and where to turn in the event of unfair treatment by an insurance company or provider.

3. Find out what medical expenses are deductible from your federal and state tax returns.

4. In the event of incapacitation, ensure your rights with an advance health care directive.

5. Use governmental agencies, consumer groups, and other sources of information to keep abreast of changes in your rights.

15

Prepare for Emergencies

No one is safe from medical emergencies such as an accident or a sudden illness, so it behooves you to prepare for them in advance of their occurrence. Medical emergencies are usually disorienting and traumatic experiences, during which time it is difficult to focus on much more than their immediate resolution.

In general, preparation for medical emergencies involves the protection of your health interests. Murphy's Law suggests that preparing for a medical emergency will actually lessen the chance of one taking place. A little planning goes a long way toward eliminating the panic and confusion that accompany a crisis situation involving your health or the health of someone you love.

Basic Preparation

One of the first tasks to prepare for a medical emergency is to be sure that all emergency contact numbers are accessible. Have on hand one of the many comprehensive guides available in bookstores that describe how to treat household accidents and other minor injuries. Keep emergency medical kits in your home and car, and know basic first aid for cuts and scrapes, burns, choking, and bleeding.

Emergency medical kits should include the following basic items:

adhesive bandages	rubbing alcohol
adhesive tape	thermometer
sterile gauze pads	hydrocortisone cream
cotton pads	tweezers
cotton swabs	petroleum jelly
smelling salts	scissors
antiseptic ointment	burn salve
instant ice packs	safety pins
hydrogen peroxide	pain relievers
disposable latex gloves	flashlight & batteries

You can also create a kit of common alternative remedies and herbs to treat minor injuries and ailments. There are prepackaged kits of homeopathic remedies, such as arnica and Rescue Remedy™, that are useful in emergencies. You can purchase these products at many locations including health food stores or directly from manufacturers. You can also have a qualified herbal specialist or homeopath custom design an emergency herbal kit for you.

Relationships to Have in Place

There are two relationships you should have in place prior to any medical emergency. A relationship with a primary care provider whom you know and trust is critical in a health crisis. Ideally, this relationship has developed over time into one that is both positive and collaborative. When you are in the midst of an emergency, you simply will not have the time or resources to search for a new provider. Even if you find one, he may not be skilled and will be limited in his ability to help you because he knows you in no other context of your life.

The second relationship you need in place prior to a medical emergency is a health care advocate, which was discussed in the previous chapter. The most important role of a health care advocate is to act in your best interests in the event of physical or emotional incapacitation, ensuring that your wishes are carried out in the manner in which you intend.

A health care advocate can accompany you to appointments, research health issues, help you to make decisions about treatment, intercede on your behalf with health professionals, and do anything that you would normally do for yourself. He can manage medications for you—how often to take them and the proper dose. An advocate can also deal with problems that arise and provide you with an emotional anchor during a very difficult time. An advocate can be particularly helpful in the time-consuming task of researching alternative medicine options.

A spouse, family member, or close friend are all good candidates for a health care advocate. Sometimes, a private-duty nurse or professional caregiver can also perform this role. An advocate should be a person who is trustworthy and willing to exercise his prerogative by placing your needs and wishes above all other concerns. Again, a health care advocate is typically designated in an advance health care directive.

Advance Health Care Directive

As outlined in the previous chapter, an advance health care directive is usually a legal document like a living will, living trust, or health care power of attorney, which details your wishes for prolonging or sustaining your life with medical intervention and for resuscitation from cardiac or respiratory arrest known as a DNR (Do Not Resuscitate) order. In some states, a living will that specifies your wishes for life-sustaining medical treatment is also termed a *declaration*.

Advance health care directives can be drawn up by an attorney or on your own, but they must comply with state law in order to be legally upheld. These documents should be witnessed and notarized by a notary public.

Having an advance health care directive can be critical in the presence of a medical emergency. A good example of this is the case in Florida where the spouse and parents of a woman in a permanent vegetative state waged a legal and legislative battle against one another for years about whether to keep her alive. An advance health care directive would have prevented this dispute. The point is that you do not want family members, let alone the courts or state government, battling over your life and guessing your intentions.

Health Care Rights

You should know your health care rights in advance of a medical emergency. Having a clear understanding of the terms and benefits of your health insurance policy, an agent who will advocate on your behalf with the insurance company, and a list of agencies offering consumer assistance are all important ways to avert problems during a medical crisis. You should know your tax rights regarding medical care and the name of an attorney who specializes in consumer law in the event your rights are violated.

Although there is no absolute right to health care, every person is entitled to certain health care rights, also addressed in the previous chapter. Health care rights vary significantly from state to state on such issues as confidentiality and access to medical records. Knowing your rights makes you feel less helpless and more empowered during a medical emergency.

Dealing with Hospitals

Medical emergencies sometimes result in the need to receive inpatient care from a hospital. Even though there is access to telephones and contact with family members and friends during hospital visiting hours, your options for investigation and treatment are severely limited until your condition is sufficiently stabilized for you to be released and go elsewhere. If you are mentally alert and have access to a laptop computer with a wireless connection, you can research health information on your own and connect with others via the Internet.

Many hospitals now employ *hospitalists*. Hospitalists are generalist physicians and internists who specialize in managing the care of inpatients, helping to reduce the stress and confusion that accompany inpatient treatment. A health care advocate can also do this but without the inside contacts and medical training. Some hospitals have advocacy programs to assist inpatients. However, hospitalists and hospital advocates can be biased about your care because, as employees of the hospital, their loyalty is ultimately to their employer, not to you. A health care advocate does not have this conflict of interest.

Although hospitals are intimidating places to be, do not be afraid to assert yourself when you are in one. Ask questions about anything you do not understand. Set limits for hospital personnel, such as requesting that you not be disturbed during the night unless medically necessary. Request copies of diagnostic tests that are ordered by your treating physician, and get copies of all paperwork that you are asked to sign. Before undergoing surgery or any invasive treatment or test, confirm your name, blood type, and procedure with the surgeon and his surgical staff. Ask for written instructions on follow-up care before leaving the hospital. Treat hospital personnel the same way you would any health provider, and expect the same standard of service and excellence from them.

Remember that the majority of hospitals are in business to make money and, as such, may try to sell you optional services that you do not want or need. When you are in a hospital, you may be visited by counseling and nutritional consultants and charged for unsolicited visits as "consultations" even if you decline the service. If you do not want a service or to be charged for an unsolicited consultation, inform the representative to avoid confusion later.

Prepare for Emergencies

Hospitals are also notorious for duplication and waste. It has been reported that there is an estimated $1,400 in overcharges on every hospital bill. Even non-profit hospitals that engage in charitable work and cater to the uninsured have been accused of overcharging customers. Since you may be required to pay a percentage or all of these charges, keep a watchful eye on your treatment and question unauthorized or unknown charges on your bill when you receive it. Reputable hospitals will usually remove questionable charges upon request.

Do not tolerate insensitive or rude hospital personnel under any circumstances. If any member of the hospital staff is unkind to you, tell your treating physician and insist that the person be replaced. There should be zero tolerance for unwarranted negative behavior in hospitals or any health care environment. Hospital personnel are there to serve you and comply with any reasonable request.

In the event of a harmful outcome from a hospital service or treatment, contact the *patient safety officer* if there is one on staff and request an honest explanation of the cause. If it is accredited by the Joint Commission on Accreditation of Healthcare Organizations (JCAHO), the hospital is required to provide this to you.

The following recapitulates recommended *Hospital Do's* and *Don'ts*:

Hospital Do's

- Do get copies of all paperwork—admitting forms, contracts for service, labwork, x-ray reports, and follow-up care.

- Do find an advocate to intercede on your behalf with hospital staff—primary care physician, patient relations representative, hospital advocate, hospitalist, spouse, family member, or friend.

- Do insist on the hospital staff catering to your needs rather than the other way around.

- Do examine your hospital bill for overcharges.

- Do demand an honest explanation if something goes wrong with your care.

Hospital Don'ts

- Don't sign anything without reading it thoroughly.

- Don't pay for services that you refuse or did not authorize.

- Don't tolerate rude or unkind behavior on the part of hospital staff.

- Don't make decisions regarding your care without knowing all of your options, including those the hospital does not offer.

There are many consumer guides that address problems associated with health care. *Take This Book to the Hospital with You* by Charles Inlander and Ed Weiner is one of the few books that specifically addresses care received in a hospital. Consumer-oriented health care books such as *The Activist Cancer Patient* by Beverly Zakarian and *The New Way*

Prepare for Emergencies

to Take Charge of Your Medical Treatment by Barbara Hardt and Katherine Halkin also provide helpful information about hospitals.

Information about hospitals is provided by the Joint Commission on Accreditation of Healthcare Organizations (JCAHO) at (603) 792-5000 or online at www.jcaho.org. For a small fee, they will send you a hospital performance report along with guidelines on choosing quality health care organizations. Hospitals that are members of the nonprofit Joint Commission for the Accreditation of Hospitals (JCAH) submit to a voluntary review of their facilities. Complaints about members should be directed to the complaint hotline at (800) 994-6610 or to the Joint Commission, Office of Quality Monitoring, One Renaissance Boulevard, Oakbrook Terrace, Illinois, 60181. Members of the American Hospital Association (AHA) must post the AHA Bill of Rights of 1973 in their facility, so it is clearly visible to consumers.

A sincere desire to be actively involved in the health care process is the greatest tool you can have to survive any medical emergency. This includes a willingness to educate yourself about health issues, take responsibility for those aspects of health over which you can exercise some control, be aware of what is transpiring around you, and make informed decisions about your care. Once these tools are in place, a medical emergency is much easier to manage and becomes much less alarming.

☑ Check List:

1. Maintain an emergency medical kit, and keep emergency phone numbers handy.

2. Develop a positive relationship with a primary care provider.

3. Select a health care advocate.

4. Establish an advance health care directive.

5. Know your health care rights.

6. Use hospitals to your benefit, not to your detriment.

16

Conclusion

There are a multitude of reasons why health care fails to meet the needs of consumers, including:

- a health care system inexorably tied to and driven by economics
- an emphasis on intervention rather than prevention
- assembly line treatment regardless of individual needs
- a lack of consideration for all aspects of health at one time—physical, emotional, and spiritual

- providers who are more focused on themselves than their patients
- patients who are disempowered by the system and not willing to take more responsibility for their health
- the existence of third-party payers or insurance companies

As the industry struggles with complicated growing pains, consumers are caught right in the middle of the struggle. Many people now find themselves in a "sink or swim" situation in health care, imprisoned by a system that has become inadequate and insensitive to their needs. Ambivalent until we have a bad experience or become seriously ill, we justify the mediocrity of our health care system by claiming that there is nothing better anywhere else in the world. This complacent attitude is exactly what keeps it both inadequate and unchanged.

Our health care system is simply not conducive to consumers getting the best care. There have been many suggestions on fixing it short of abolishing it and starting over, which is probably what we should do if we really want it to be truly responsive to our needs. Many people believe that government-sponsored, national health care is the answer, doing away with health plans altogether. Others suggest that adapting information technologies on a widespread basis will alleviate some of the problems.

Everyone agrees that regulators should be held accountable for their actions, but others point out that hospitals, providers, and manufacturers of health products should be too. Consumer groups insist that substandard providers be identified and retrained before they cause more harm. These

Conclusion

groups want to publish information about them, so people can decide for themselves where and from whom they want to receive care.

The problem is that these changes will only improve health care to a certain point, if they do at all. They omit the most important aspect of improved health care—an active, fully involved, and empowered health care consumer. There are several realities we must consider in assuming this role:

- *Health care has become more complicated than it needs to be or should be.* It is much simpler than providers, science, technology, insurance companies, and governments have made it for us.

- *Maintaining or achieving health is more complex than we think it should be, involving more than taking a pill or having a single treatment.* Although being well was always complicated, it is even more so today with the accumulation of man-made threats to our health that did not exist fifty years ago.

- *People know much more about what they need in order to achieve and maintain health than those in the health care system would have us believe.* We only need to develop the skills that allow us to make these determinations. There is no way to get better care without our doing this and no short cut to this process.

Other realities loom in our path. There is more health information available to us as consumers than ever before. But the information is overwhelming, frequently contradictory, and subject to constant revision, and a sizable portion of it is downright unreliable. We also have more awareness than ever before about the need to simplify our lives, yet we continue to allow them to become more and more complicated. We know what it takes to be healthy but have less time, money, and inclination to achieve it; it just seems like too much work to do what is necessary to be well. And we are programmed to abdicate power to those who are supposed to serve us, paying a heavy price for it in the process.

Money and power, the cornerstones of a capitalistic society, create a culture of permission, and nowhere is this more evident than in the health care industry. Regulators deny necessary care to save money but spend millions of dollars defeating legislation that would empower you and your provider. Providers perform unnecessary procedures to make money but spend millions of dollars preventing you from finding out who among them are the bad apples. Hospitals make avoidable mistakes and then try to cover them up to avoid compensating those they have harmed with their errors. Pharmaceutical companies charge exorbitant prices for drugs sold at one-half the price in other countries and mislead consumers about their adverse effects. It takes a lot of courage and perseverance to overcome the negativity of health care in our society today.

It seems as though there is very little we can do to change our health care system because it has become so big and powerful. It would be easy to regard the recommendations in this guide as a futile attempt to make the best of a very bad situation that only seems to be getting worse every day. Although we have little control over what politicians, insurance companies, providers, hospitals, and drug companies do, we do have control over what we do and how we deal with them. This is the one thing we *can* change.

Conclusion

The only way to change the system is to change ourselves and our role in the system. We can accomplish this in three ways:

1. *Do everything possible to protect yourself,* which is the basis for the twelve steps outlined in this book. Although there is no guarantee of a positive outcome from any health care service or product, performing these steps will greatly increase your chances of receiving one.

2. *If you are seriously injured by the negligence or incompetence of a health care provider, take action to ensure that the behavior is not repeated with others.* Although your efforts may not yield immediate results or the appropriate punishment, putting it on record is cathartic and will be more difficult for authorities to ignore the second time around.

3. *After you have taken appropriate action, find something positive about the experience, no matter how small or seemingly insignificant, so you can let go of the anger and move on.* For example, what did you learn from the experience? Have you become a more patient or compassionate person as a result of the experience?

Achieving health is a reachable goal if you are truly willing to take responsibility for your physical, emotional, and spiritual well-being. You will get more out of the medicine you are using, conventional or alternative, if you are more involved in your own care. Performing the tasks outlined in this guide will help you to accomplish this goal with a minimum of effort but a maximum of benefit. They can be applied to any type of care—outpatient or inpatient and preventive or therapeutic.

Taking the steps recommended in this guide sounds easy in theory but may be more difficult in practice. Educating yourself about health issues, changing attitudes and behaviors that impede your ability to get the most from any medicine, and initiating the appropriate action can be an intimidating and time-consuming process.

As a result of this, you should not feel compelled to perform all of these tasks at once. Performing one or two steps well is better than performing all of them poorly or doing nothing at all. Most people wait for serious illness to strike before they are motivated to be more actively involved in their own care. If you wait until that happens, it will be too late to effect any real change when you need it the most.

Many people question the benefits of becoming more educated in a system of medicine that is not only autocratic but also very confusing and rightly so. Every provider has a different opinion about what to do, and medical science changes its mind with each new study. In other words, becoming more educated in our system of medicine is analogous to becoming less certain about what to do. The reason this is such a problem is because we rely way too much on the opinions of others and the results of scientific studies to determine our choices.

The most important task in becoming a better health care consumer is to begin to listen to yourself and trust that you know or have the power to determine the right course of action. You can use this knowledge to consider all your options and choose the right one for you. Listening to yourself is about mental and spiritual awareness and growth. It provides inner strength and guidance and can be realized in many ways. You must choose the path that works best for you and fits into your lifestyle, values, beliefs, and worldview.

Conclusion

There are many books, available at your local bookstore, that are exclusively devoted to developing this natural ability.

When you assume a more active role, you must also be prepared for resistance from health professionals. Resistant providers may try to rein you in by telling you, "There is a problem with people who want to manage their own care" or "Patients cannot know more than their doctors." Providers may become uncooperative, defensive, or even unfriendly toward you. When you take on an entrenched medical establishment in this manner, you also risk being labeled a "difficult patient."

There really is such a thing as a difficult patient because, as we all know, there are difficult people. The definition of this label, however, has unfairly broadened over the years to include any person who asserts himself in the health care process. Likewise, the definition of the "good patient" has unfairly narrowed to apply only to those who dutifully comply with a provider's wishes.

Do not be discouraged from taking a more active role by such disparaging remarks or disapproving labels. You must be impervious to negativity and any attempts to dissuade you from becoming more involved in your own care. If being a difficult patient is defined as refusing to relinquish your authority as a responsible health care consumer, you should consider this label a supreme compliment.

Good patients not only assume an active role in their own care and treatment, but they are also willing to take charge of all aspects of their health, doing so safely, effectively, and responsibly. As long as you are reasonable in your expectations and demands, responsible providers will respect rather than resent you for your involvement. It ultimately makes their job easier and improves your chances for good health.

Resistance from health professionals can actually be advantageous to you. In the presence of this obstacle, you are often jolted into realizing exactly what you want and who you want to provide it to you. Initial resistence from a provider does not necessarily mean that he should be immediately replaced. Like anything new, your new role takes getting used to on both sides of the fence. You can encourage the process by making changes gradually. Gradual change gives everyone the time to adjust and reduces the risk of a negative response or outcome.

Becoming a better health care consumer has the power to transform not only your health but also your experience with health care. The system improves because the participants have the opportunity to witness firsthand the positive effect you have on your own care. With more effective consumerism, providers benefit from fewer mistakes and better health outcomes and regulators benefit from reduced costs. Since our health care system has become so complex with such potential for harm, your active involvement is necessary not only to improve the system but to survive it.

Blind faith about health and blind trust toward health care are luxuries we can no longer afford. Attitudes like these are as ridiculous as performing no maintenance on a car until it breaks down or buying a new house without first performing inspections, only with far greater consequences. Without health, our options are extremely limited.

When you become a better health care consumer, you receive the best possible care. The best possible care results in a better outcome from the health care service. When you

Conclusion

enjoy a better outcome from the health care service, you have a better chance to maintain or improve your health. The result of maintaining or improving your health is a better and longer life.

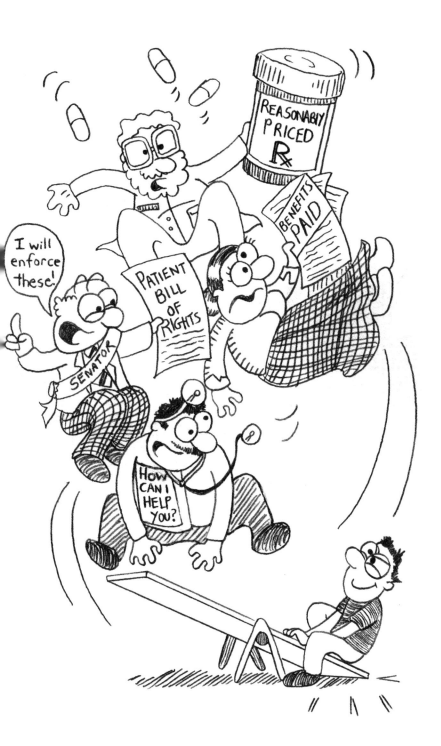

To defy Power, which seems omnipotent; . . .
This is alone Life; . . .

PERCY SHELLEY
Prometheus Unbound (1820)

APPENDIX

A

State Agencies & Licensing Boards

Please note that each state government maintains a website with listings of additional agencies and boards. You can also consult the state government listing of your local telephone directory.

Alabama (334)

Information	242–8000
Dept of Health	206–5300
Mental Health	242–3454
Consumer Protect	242–7334
Insurance Dept	269–3550
Licensing:	
Dentists	(205) 985–7267
Nurses	242–4060
Physicians	242–4116

Alaska (907)

Information	465–2111
Dept of Health	465–3030
Mental Health	465–3370
Consumer Protect	465–2133
Insurance Dept	465–2515
Licensing:	
Dentists	465–2542
Nurses	269–8161
Physicians	269–8163
Other	465–2534

Arizona (602)

Information	542–4900
Dept of Health	542–1000
Mental Health	364–4558
Consumer Protect	542–5763
Insurance Dept	912–8400
Licensing:	
Dentists	242–1492
Nurses	331–8111
Physicians	551–2700
Osteopaths	657–7703
Other	364–3526

Arkansas (501)

Information	682–3000
Dept of Health	661–2000
Mental Health	686–9164
Consumer Protect	682–6150
Insurance Dept	371–2600
Licensing:	
Dentists	682–2085
Nurses	686–2700
Physicians	296–1802

California (916)

Information	657–9900
Dept of Health	445–4171
Mental Health	654–3565
Consumer Protect	445–1254
Insurance Dept	492–3500
Licensing:	
Dentists	263–2300
Nurses	322–3350
Physicians	263–2382
Osteopaths	263–3100

Colorado (303)

Information	866–5000
Dept of Health	692–2035
Mental Health	866–7400
Consumer Protect	866–5189
Insurance Dept	894–7499
Licensing:	
Dentists	894–7761
Nurses	894–2430
Physicians	894–7690
Other	894–7855

State Agencies & Licensing Boards

Connecticut (860)

Information	566–2211
Dept of Health	418–7000
Mental Health	509–8045
Consumer Protect	713–6020
Insurance Dept	297–3800
Licensing:	
Dentists	509–7648
Nurses	509–7624
Physicians	509–7643
Osteopaths	509–7563
Other	509–7603

Delaware (302)

Information	739–4000
Dept of Health	255–9040
Mental Health	255–9399
Consumer Protect	577–8600
Insurance Dept	739–4251
Licensing:	
Dentists	744–4518
Nurses	577–3288
Physicians	744–4507
Other	744–4500

District of Columbia (202)

Information	727–1000
Dept of Health	442–5999
Mental Health	673–7440
Consumer Protect	442–4400
Insurance Dept	727–8000
Licensing:	
Dentists	442–4764
Nurses	442–4776
Physicians	442–9200
Other	442–9200

Florida (850)

Information	488–1234
Dept of Health	245–4321
Mental Health	487–1111
Consumer Protect	922–2966
Insurance Dept	922–3132
Licensing:	
Dentists	245–4474
Nurses	245–4125
Physicians	245–4131
Osteopaths	414–1976
Other	488–0595

Georgia (404)

Information	656–2000
Dept of Health	657–2700
Mental Health	657–2270
Consumer Protect	656–3790
Insurance Dept	656–2056

Licensing:

Dentists	(478) 207–1680
Nurses	(478) 207–1640
Physicians	656–3913
Other	207–1686

Hawaii (808)

Information	586–2211
Dept of Health	586–4400
Mental Health	586–4686
Consumer Protect	586–2630
Insurance Dept	586–2790

Licensing:

Dentists	586–2702
Nurses	586–2695
Physicians	586–2708
Other	586–3000

Idaho (208)

Information	334–2411
Dept of Health	334–5500
Mental Health	334–5528
Consumer Protect	334–2424
Insurance Dept	334–4250

Licensing:

Dentists	334–2369
Nurses	334–3110
Physicians	327–7000
Other	334–3233

Illinois (217)

Information	782–2000
Dept of Health	782–4977
Mental Health	557–1601
Consumer Protect	814–3000
Insurance Dept	782–4515

Licensing:

Dentists	782–0458
Nurses	782–0458
Physicians	782–0458
Other	782–0458

State Agencies & Licensing Boards

Indiana (317)

Information	232–1000
Dept of Health	233–1325
Mental Health	232–7800
Consumer Protect	232–6330
Insurance Dept	232–2385

Licensing:

Dentists	234–2057
Nurses	234–2043
Physicians	234–2060
Other	232–2980

Iowa (515)

Information	281–5011
Dept of Health	281–5787
Mental Health	281–5874
Consumer Protect	281–5926
Insurance Dept	281–5705

Licensing:

Dentists	281–5157
Nurses	281–3255
Physicians	281–5171
Other	281–4287

Kansas (785)

Information	296–0111
Dept of Health	296–1086
Mental Health	296–3773
Consumer Protect	296–3751
Insurance Dept	296–3071

Licensing:

Dentists	296–6400
Nurses	296–4929
Physicians	296–7413
Other	296–7413

Kentucky (502)

Information	564–2500
Dept of Health	564–3970
Mental Health	564–3844
Consumer Protect	696–5389
Insurance Dept	564–3630

Licensing:

Dentists	423–0573
Nurses	329–7000
Physicians	429–8046
Other	564–3296

Louisiana (255)

Information	342–6600
Dept of Health	342–9500
Mental Health	342–2540
Consumer Protect	342–7186
Insurance Dept	342–5900

Licensing:

Dentists	568–8574
Nurses	838–5332
Physicians	568–6820
Other	342–9500

Maine (207)

Information	624–9494
Dept of Health	287–8016
Mental Health	287–4200
Consumer Protect	626–8000
Insurance Dept	624–8475

Licensing:

Dentists	287–3333
Nurses	287–1133
Physicians	287–3601
Osteopaths	287–2480
Other	624–8500

Maryland (410)

Information	634–6361
Dept of Health	767–6860
Mental Health	402–8300
Consumer Protect	528–8662
Insurance Dept	468–2000

Licensing:

Dentists	402–8500
Nurses	585–1900
Physicians	764–4777
Other	764–4700

Massachusetts (617)

Information	727–2121
Dept of Health	624–6000
Mental Health	626–8000
Consumer Protect	727–2200
Insurance Dept	468–2000

Licensing:

Dentists	727–9928
Nurses	727–9961
Physicians	654–9800
Other	727–3074

State Agencies & Licensing Boards

Michigan (517)

Information	373–1837
Dept of Health	373–0408
Mental Health	373–3500
Consumer Protect	727–2200
Insurance Dept	373–9273

Licensing:

Dentists	335–1752
Nurses	373–1600
Physicians	373–6873
Other	241–9427

Minnesota (651)

Information	296–6013
Dept of Health	215–5800
Mental Health	296–6045
Consumer Protect	296–3353
Insurance Dept	297–7161

Licensing:

Dentists	617–2250
Nurses	617–2270
Physicians	617–2130
Other	282–6366

Mississippi (601)

Information	359–1000
Dept of Health	576–7400
Mental Health	359–1288
Consumer Protect	359–1100
Insurance Dept	359–3569

Licensing:

Dentists	944–9622
Nurses	987–4188
Physicians	987–3079
Other	576–8064

Missouri (573)

Information	751–2000
Dept of Health	751–6400
Mental Health	751–4122
Consumer Protect	751–3321
Insurance Dept	751–4126

Licensing:

Dentists	751–0040
Nurses	751–0681
Physicians	751–0098
Other	751–0293

Montana (406)

Information	444–2511
Dept of Health	444–5622
Mental Health	444–3964
Consumer Protect	444–3553
Insurance Dept	444–2047

Licensing:

Dentists	841–2390
Nurses	841–2340
Physicians	841–2363
Other	841–2300

Nebraska (402)

Information	471–2311
Dept of Health	471–3121
Mental Health	479–5166
Consumer Protect	471–2682
Insurance Dept	471–2201

Licensing:

Dentists	471–2118
Nurses	471–4921
Physicians	471–2118
Other	471–2133

Nevada (775)

Information	687–5000
Dept of Health	684–4200
Mental Health	684–5943
Consumer Protect	486–7355
Insurance Dept	687–4270

Licensing:

Dentists	486–7044
Nurses	688–2620
Physicians	688–2559
Osteopaths	(702) 732–2147
Other	684–4475

New Hampshire (603)

Information	271–1110
Dept of Health	271–4685
Mental Health	271–5000
Consumer Protect	271–3641
Insurance Dept	271–2261

Licensing:

Dentists	271–4561
Nurses	271–2323
Physicians	271–1203
Other	271–4814

State Agencies & Licensing Boards

New Jersey (609)

Information	292–2121
Dept of Health	292–7837
Mental Health	777–0700
Consumer Protect	504–6200
Insurance Dept	292–5360
Licensing:	
Dentists	(973) 504–6405
Nurses	504–6430
Physicians	826–7100
Other	504–6200

New Mexico (505)

Information	827–9632
Dept of Health	827–2613
Mental Health	827–2601
Consumer Protect	827–6060
Insurance Dept	827–4297
Licensing:	
Dentists	476–7125
Nurses	841–8340
Physicians	827–5022
Osteopaths	476–7120
Other	827–7003

New York (518)

Information	474–2121
Dept of Health	474–2011
Mental Health	474–6540
Consumer Protect	474–1471
Insurance Dept	474–6600
Licensing:	
Dentists	474–3817
Nurses	474–3817
Physicians	474–3817
Other	474–3817

North Carolina (919)

Information	733–1110
Dept of Health	733–4534
Mental Health	733–7011
Consumer Protect	716–6000
Insurance Dept	733–7343
Licensing:	
Dentists	678–8223
Nurses	782–3211
Physicians	326–1100
Other	807–2000

North Dakota (701)

Information	328–2000
Dept of Health	328–2372
Mental Health	328–2310
Consumer Protect	328–3404
Insurance Dept	224–2440
Licensing:	
Dentists	258–8600
Nurses	328–9777
Physicians	328–6500
Other	328–2219

Ohio (614)

Information	466–2000
Dept of Health	466–2253
Mental Health	466–2596
Consumer Protect	466–8831
Insurance Dept	644–2658
Licensing:	
Dentists	466–2580
Nurses	466–6940
Physicians	466–3934
Other	466–8734

Oklahoma (405)

Information	521–2011
Dept of Health	271–4200
Mental Health	522–3878
Consumer Protect	522–0085
Insurance Dept	521–2828
Licensing:	
Dentists	524–9037
Nurses	962–1800
Physicians	848–6841
Osteopaths	528–8625
Other	848–6841

Oregon (503)

Information	378–6500
Dept of Health	731–4000
Mental Health	945–5763
Consumer Protect	378–4100
Insurance Dept	947–7984
Licensing:	
Dentists	229–5520
Nurses	731–4745
Physicians	229–5770
Other	378–8667

State Agencies & Licensing Boards

Pennsylvania (717)

Information	787–2121
Dept of Health	783–5685
Mental Health	787–6443
Consumer Protect	783–5048
Insurance Dept	787–5173
Licensing:	
Dentists	783–7162
Nurses	783–7142
Physicians	783–1400
Osteopaths	783–4858
Other	787–8503

Rhode Island (401)

Information	222–2000
Dept of Health	222–2231
Mental Health	462–3201
Consumer Protect	277–4400
Insurance Dept	222–2246
Licensing:	
Dentists	277–2827
Nurses	222–5700
Physicians	222–3855
Other	222–6015

South Carolina (803)

Information	896–0000
Dept of Health	898–3432
Mental Health	898–8581
Consumer Protect	734–4200
Insurance Dept	737–6160
Licensing:	
Dentists	896–4599
Nurses	896–4550
Physicians	896–4500
Other	896–4300

South Dakota (605)

Information	773–3011
Dept of Health	773–3361
Mental Health	773–5991
Consumer Protect	773–4400
Insurance Dept	773–4104
Licensing:	
Dentists	224–1282
Nurses	362–2760
Physicians	336–1965
Other	773–3361

Tennessee (615)

Information	741–3011
Dept of Health	741–3111
Mental Health	532–6610
Consumer Protect	741–4737
Insurance Dept	741–2241
Licensing:	
Dentists	532–5073
Nurses	532–5166
Physicians	532–3202
Other	741–8402

Texas (512)

Information	463–4630
Dept of Health	458–7111
Mental Health	454–3761
Consumer Protect	463–2185
Insurance Dept	463–6169
Licensing:	
Dentists	463–6400
Nurses	305–7400
Physicians	305–7030
Other	834–6628

Utah (801)

Information	538–3000
Dept of Health	538–6111
Mental Health	538–4270
Consumer Protect	530–6601
Insurance Dept	530–3800
Licensing:	
Dentists	530–6767
Nurses	530–6628
Physicians	530–6628
Other	530–6628

Vermont (802)

Information	828–1110
Dept of Health	863–7200
Mental Health	241–2100
Consumer Protect	656–3183
Insurance Dept	828–3301
Licensing:	
Dentists	828–2390
Nurses	828–2396
Physicians	657–4220
Osteopath	828–2373
Other	828–2363

State Agencies & Licensing Boards

Virginia (804)

Information	786–0000
Dept of Health	786–3561
Mental Health	786–3921
Consumer Protect	786–2043
Insurance Dept	371–9741
Licensing:	
Dentists	662–9906
Nurses	662–9909
Physicians	662–9908
Other	662–9900

Washington (360)

Information	753–5000
Dept of Health	236–4010
Mental Health	902–8070
Consumer Protect	753–6210
Insurance Dept	753–7300
Licensing:	
Dentists	236–4863
Nurses	236–4700
Physicians	236–4788
Osteopaths	236–4945
Other	236–4700

West Virginia (304)

Information	558–3456
Dept of Health	558–2971
Mental Health	558–0627
Consumer Protect	558–8986
Insurance Dept	558–3354
Licensing:	
Dentists	252–8266
Nurses	558–3596
Physicians	558–2921
Osteopaths	723–4638

Wisconsin (608)

Information	266–2211
Dept of Health	266–1865
Mental Health	266–1351
Consumer Protect	224–4960
Insurance Dept	266–3585
Licensing:	
Dentists	266–0483
Nurses	266–0145
Physicians	266–2112
Other	266–2112

Wyoming (307)

Information	777–7220
Dept of Health	777–7656
Mental Health	777–7094
Consumer Protect	777–7874
Insurance Dept	777–7401
Licensing:	
Dentists	777–6529
Nurses	777–7601
Physicians	777–7053
Other	777–7378

Puerto Rico (787)

Dept of Health	274–7604
Mental Health	764–7855
Consumer Protect	721–0940
Insurance Dept	722–8686
Licensing:	
Dentists	723–1617
Nurses	725–7506
Physicians	782–8989

Virgin Islands (340)

Information	778–0997
Dept of Health	773–1311
Mental Health	773–1992
Consumer Protect	773–2226
Insurance Dept	773–6449
Licensing:	
Dentists	774–0117
Nurses	776–7397
Physicians	774–0117

APPENDIX B

Consumer Advocacy Groups, Health Rights Organizations & Medical Information Services

Consumer Advocacy Groups

Campaign for Environmentally Responsible Health Care (202) 234–9121
Center for Medical Consumers (212) 674–7105
Citizen's Council on Health Care (651) 646–8935
Citizens For Health (202) 483–4344
Committee For Freedom Of Choice In Medicine (800) 227–4473 or (619) 429–8200
Consumer's Union (914) 378–2000
National Women's Health Network (202) 628–7814
Public Citizen Health Research Group (202) 588–1000

Health Rights Organizations

American Civil Liberties Union (ACLU) (212) 549–2500 (check local listings for state chapters)
Center for Health Care Rights (213) 383–4519 or (800) 824–0780
Citizens Council on Health Care (651) 646–8935
Electronic Privacy Information Center (202) 483–1140
Foundation for Taxpayer and Consumer Rights (310) 392–0522
Health Privacy Project/Institute for Health Care Research and Policy (202) 721–5632
National Coalition for Patient Rights (207) 774–8800
Patient Advocate Foundation (800) 532–5274

Medical Information Services

Can Help (360) 437–2291 (specifically for cancer)
Health Resource (800) 949–0090 or (501) 329–5272
Medical Information Foundation (800) 999–1999 or (650) 326–6000
Planetree Foundation (415) 923–3680
Schine Online Services (800) 346–3287 or (401) 751–3320
World Research Foundation (928) 284–3300

APPENDIX

C

Professional Associations & Organizations

CONVENTIONAL MEDICINE

Conventional Medicine—General

American Board of Medical Specialties (866) 275–2267
American College of Surgeons (312) 202–5000
American Medical Association (312) 464–5000
American Medical Women's Association (703) 838–0500
American Nurses Association (202) 651–7000 or (800) 274–4262
National Association Medical Staff Services (512) 454–7928
Society for the Advancement of Women's Health Research (202) 223–8224

Conventional Medicine—Miscellaneous

American Association of Nutritional Consultants (888) 828–2262
American Dental Association (312) 440–2500
American Dietetic Association (800) 877–1600
American Hospital Association (312) 422–3000
Joint Commission on Accreditation of Healthcare Organizations (603) 792–5000
Nutrition Education Association (713) 665–2946
Society of Certified Nutritionists (800) 342–8037

Psychotherapy

American Association for Marriage and Family Therapy (202) 452–0109
American Counseling Association (703) 823–9800 or (800) 347–6647
American Psychiatric Association (703) 907–7300
American Psychological Association (202) 336–5500 or (800) 374–2721
Association for Humanistic Psychology (510) 769–6495
Association for Transpersonal Psychology (650) 424–8764
International Association of Counselors and Therapists (941) 498–9710
International Somatic Movement Education and Therapy Association (212) 229–7666
National Association of Social Workers (202) 408–8600
Society for Spirituality and Social Work (607) 777–4603
U.S. Association for Body Psychotherapy (202) 446–1619

Professional Associations & Organizations

ALTERNATIVE MEDICINE

Alternative Medicine—General

American Association for Health Freedom (800) 230–2762
American Board of Holistic Medicine (808) 572–4616
American Holistic Health Association (714) 779–6152
American Holistic Medical Association (505) 292–7788
American Holistic Nurses Association (800) 278–2462
American Holistic Veterinary Medical Association (410) 569–0795
Complementary-Alternative Medical Association (404) 284–7592
Holistic Dental Association (970) 259–109
National Center for Complementary and Alternative Medicine (NIH) (301) 519–3153 or (888) 644–6226
National Wellness Institute (715) 342–2969 or (800) 243–8694
National Women's Health Network (202) 347–1140
Society of Behavioral Medicine (608) 827–7267

Alternative Medicine—Miscellaneous

American Academy of Anti-Aging Medicine (773) 528–4333
American Academy of Environmental Medicine (316) 684–5500
American Academy of Pain Management (209) 533–9744
American Association for Music Therapy (301) 589–3300
American Board of Chelation Therapy (800) 356–2228
Association for Applied Psychophysiology and Biofeedback (303) 422–8436 or (800) 477–8892
Biofeedback Certification Institute of America (303) 420–2902
Institute of Noetic Sciences (707) 775–3500
International Association for Colon Hydrotherapy (210) 366–2888
International Association for Oxygen Therapy (208) 448–2504
International Society for the Study of Subtle Energies and Energy Medicine (303) 425–4625

Is Your Health Care Killing You?

Midwives' Alliance of North America (888) 923–6262
Society for Light Treatment and Biological Rhythms
(415) 751–2758 Fax

Bodywork

American Academy of Reflexology (818) 841–7741
American Massage Therapy Association (847) 864–0123
American Organization for Bodywork Therapies of Asia
(856) 782–1616
American Oriental Bodywork Therapy Association
(856) 782–1616
American Polarity Therapy Association (303) 545–2080
American Society for the Alexander Technique (413) 584–2359 or (800) 473–0620
Associated Bodywork and Massage Professionals
(800) 458–2267
Federation of Therapeutic Massage, Bodywork and Somatic
Practice Organizations (847) 864–0123
Feldenkrais Guild of North America (800) 775–2118
Hellerwork International (800) 392–3900
International Association of Reiki Professionals (603) 881–8838
International Foundation of Bio-Magnetics (520) 751–7751
International Institute of Medical Qigong (831) 646–9399
International Massage Association (540) 351–0800
International Nurses Association Complementary Therapists
(504) 893–8002
National Association of Myofascial Trigger Point Therapists
(800) 845–3454
National Certification for Therapeutic Massage and Bodywork
(800) 296–0664
Nurse Healers-Professional Associates International
(801) 273–3399
Reflexology Association of America (508) 364–4234

Professional Associations & Organizations

Rolf Institute (303) 449–5903
Trager Association (216) 896–9383

Comprehensive Systems of Alternative Medicine

Acupuncture & Oriental Medicine Alliance (253) 851–6896
American Academy of Medical Acupuncture (323) 937–5514
American Association of Ayurvedic Sciences (425) 453–8022 (medical clinic)
American Association of Naturopathic Physicians (202) 895–1392 or (866) 538–2267
American Association of Oriental Medicine (301) 941–1064 or (888) 500–7999
American Naturopathic Medical Association (702) 897–7053
Ayurveda Holistic Center and School of Ayurvedic Science (800) 452–1798.
Ayurvedic Institute (505) 291–9698
College of Maharishi Ayurveda (800) 369–6480 (instruction only)
Homeopathic Academy of Naturopathic Physicians (208) 336–9242
National Center for Homeopathy (703) 548–7790
National Certification Commission for Acupuncture and Oriental Medicine (703) 548–9004

Herbal/Plant Medicine

American Association of Naturopathic Physicians (866) 538–2267
American Botanical Council (512) 926–4900
American Herbalists Guild (770) 751–6021
American Horticulture Therapy Association (800) 634–1603
Bach Flower Essences International Education Program (800) 334–0843
Herb Research Foundation (303) 449–2265
National Association for Holistic Aromatherapy (206) 547--2164 or (888) 275–6242

Pacific Institute of Aromatherapy (415) 479–9121
World Wide Essence Society (978) 369–8454

Inward Disciplines

Aikido Association of America (773) 525–3141
American Foundation of Traditional Chinese Medicine (415) 956–3030
American Yoga Association (941) 927–4977
Insight Meditation Society (978) 355–4378
National Qigong Association (218) 365–6330
Qigong Institute (650) 323–1221
Transcendental Meditation® Program (888) 532–7686
Yoga Alliance (877) 964–2255

Mind/Body Therapies

Academy for Guided Imagery (800) 726–2070
American Association for Therapeutic Humor (602) 995–1454
American Society of Clinical Hypnosis (630) 980–4740
Association for Past-Life Research and Therapies (909) 784–1570
International Imagery Association (914) 476–0781
International Medical and Dental Hypnotherapy Association (800) 257–5467
National Guild of Hypnotists (603) 429–9438

Physical Medicine

American Academy of Osteopathy (317) 879–1881
American Chiropractic Association (703) 243–2593 or (800) 986–4636
American Osteopathic Association (800) 621–1773
International Chiropractors Association (703) 528–5000 or (800) 423–4690
International College of Applied Kinesiology (913) 384–5336

Bibliography

ABC News TV Special Report. *Bitter Medicine: Pills, Profit and the Public Health.* Hosted by Peter Jennings. May 29, 2002.

Abelson, Reed, "Drug Sales Bring Huge Profits, and Scrutiny, to Cancer Doctors," *New York Times*, January 26, 2003.

Ad Hoc Committee on Health Literacy for the Council on Scientific Affairs, American Medical Association. "Health Literacy." *Journal of American Medical Association* 281 (February 10, 1999): 552–57.

Adler, S.R., and J.R. Fosket. "Disclosing Complementary and Alternative Medicine Use in the Medical Encounter: A Qualitative Study in Women with Breast Cancer." *Journal of Family Practice* 48 (June 1999): 453–58.

American Medical Association. *Physician Characteristics and Distribution in the U.S., 2003–2004 Edition.* Chicago: AMA Press, 2003.

Arroliga, A. "A Study of Consecutive Autopsies in a Medical ICU." *Chest* 119 (2001): 530–36.

Bernstein, S.J., et al. "The Appropriateness of Hysterectomy: A comparison of Care in Seven Health Plans." *Journal of American Medical Association* 269 (May 12, 1993): 2398–2402.

Chassin, Mark R. "Assessing Strategies For Quality Improvement." *Health Affairs* 16 (May/June 1997): 151–61.

Cherry, D.K., and D.A. Woodwell. "National Ambulatory Medical Care Survey: 2000 Summary." *Advance Data From Vital and Health Statistics* No. 328. Hyattsville, Maryland: National Center for Health Statistics, June 5, 2002.

Couris, Rebecca, et al. "Medication Error Study." Boston: Massachusetts Board of Registration in Pharmacy, 1999.

Curtis, Travis C., and Sheri T. Hester. "Global Chemical Pollution." *Environmental Science & Technology* 25 (May 1991): 814–819.

Dessmon, Y.H., et al. "A Study of Consecutive Autopsies in a Medical ICU: A Comparison of Clinical Cause of Death and Autopsy Diagnosis." *CHEST* 119 (February 2001): 530–36.

Eisenberg, J.M., and A.J. Rosoff. "Physician Responsibility for the Cost of Unnecessary Medical Services." *New England Journal of Medicine* 299 (July 13, 1978): 76–80.

Eisenberg, D.M., et al. "Perceptions about Complementary Therapies Relative to Conventional Therapies among Adults Who Use Both: Results from a National Survey." *Annals of Internal Medicine* 135 (September 4, 2001): 344–51.

Elder, N., Gillcrist, A., and Minz, R. "Use of Alternative Health Care by Family Practice Patients." *Archives of Family Medicine*, American Medical Association 6 (March, 1997): 181–84.

Employment Policy Foundation. "Medical Malpractice Litigation Raises Health Care Cost, Reduces Access and Lowers Quality of Care." *Issue Backgrounder*, June 19, 2003.

Families USA. *Six Good Reasons for States to Expand Drug Coverage or Reduce Drug Prices: Background for Building an Argument.* Washington, D.C.: Families USA, November 2001.

Families USA. *Profiting from Pain: Where Prescription Drug Dollars Go.* Publication No. 02–105. Washington, D.C.: Families USA, July 2002.

Federation of Nurses and Health Professionals Survey. *The Nurse Shortage: Perspectives from Current Direct Care Nurses and Former Direct Care Nurses.* Washington, D.C.: American Federation of Teachers, April, 2001.

Bibliography

Findlay, Steve. *Prescription Drug Expenditures in 2000: The Upward Trend Continues*. Washington, D.C.: National Institute for Health Care Management Research and Education Foundation, May 8, 2001.

Fontanarosa, Phil B., Rennie Drummond, and Catherine D. DeAngelis. "Postmarketing Surveillance—Lack of Vigilance, Lack of Trust." *Journal of American Medical Association* 292 (December 1, 2004): 2647–50.

HealthFocus® International. *2001 HealthFocus® Survey*. Atlanta, Georgia: HealthFocus® International, 2001.

Heffler, Stephen, et al. for the National Health Statistics Group, Office of the Actuary, Centers for Medicare and Medicaid Services. "Health Spending Projections Through 2013," *Health Affairs*, Web Exclusive (February 11, 2004). Available from http://content.healthaffairs.org/webexclusives/index.dtl?year=2004; INTERNET.

Inlander, Charles, Interview, "Hospital Overcharge Self-Defense," *Bottom Line/Health*, April 1, 2000.

Institute for the Future. *The Future of the Internet in Health Care: Five-Year Forecast*. Oakland, California: California HealthCare Foundation, January 1999.

Institute of Medicine. *Unequal Treatment: Confronting Racial and Ethnic Disparities in Health Care*. Washington, D.C.: National Academy of Sciences Press, March 20, 2002.

Institute of Medicine. *Crossing the Quality Chasm: A New Health System for the 21st Century*. March 1, 2001.

Institute of Medicine. *Care Without Coverage: Too Little, Too Late*. National Academy of Sciences Press, May 21, 2002.

Institute of Medicine. Committee on Quality of Health Care in America. *To Err is Human: Building a Safer Health System*. Edited by Linda T. Kohn, Janet M. Corrigan, and Molla S. Donaldson. Washington, D.C.: National Academy of Sciences Press, September 1, 1999.

Institute of Medicine. *The Future of the Public's Health in the 21st Century.* National Academy of Sciences Press, November 11, 2002.

Institute for the Future. *A Forecast of Health and Health Care in America: The Future Beyond 2005.* Princeton, New Jersey: November 1998.

Jay, J.R. "Furthering Cost-effective Medical Practice." *Hospital Health Services Administration* 30 (July-Aug 1985): 65–76.

Kaiser Family Foundation. *Trends and Indicators in the Changing Health Care Marketplace, 2004 Update.* Health Care Marketplace Project, Publication No. 7031, April 2004.

Le Fever, G.B., K.V. Dawson, and A.L. Morrow. "The Extent of Drug Therapy for Attention Deficit-hyperactivity Disorder Among Children in Public Schools." *American Journal of Public Health* 89 (September 1999): 1359–64.

Mayer, Thom, and Robert Cates. "Service Excellence in Health Care." *Journal of American Medical Association* 282 (October 6, 1999): 1281–83.

McGlynn, E.A., et al. "The Quality of Health Care Delivered to Adults in the United States." *New England Journal of Medicine* 348 (June 26, 2003): 2635–45.

Nader, Ralph, Interview by David Wallis, *New York Times Magazine*, June 16, 2002.

National Institutes of Health. *Federal Obligation for Health R&D, by Source or Performer Fiscal Years 1985–2000.* Washington, D.C.: National Institutes of Health, last updated on 4/16/02. Available from http://grants1.nih.gov/grants/award/award.htm; INTERNET.

National Public Radio, Morning Edition. *Non-Profit Hospitals Care For Uninsured Scrutinized.* Reported by Julie Rovner. June 23, 2004.

Office of Inspector General, Centers for Medicare and Medicaid Services. *Inspector General's Report on the Health Care Financing Administration's Financial Statements for FY 1997.* Washington, D.C.: U.S. Department of Health and Human Services, March, 1998.

Bibliography

Ornish, D., et al. "Intensive Lifestyle Changes for Reversal of Coronary Heart Disease." *Journal of American Medical Association* 280 (December 16, 1998): 2001–7.

PBS Frontline. *Dangerous Prescription*. Written, produced, and directed by Andrew Liebman. November 13, 2003. Available from http://www.pbs.org/wgbh/pages/frontline/shows/prescription; INTERNET.

Phillips, David P., Nicholas Christenfeld, and Laura M. Glynn. "Increase in U.S. Medication-Error Deaths Between 1983 and 1993." *Lancet* 351(February 28, 1998): 643–44.

Pugh, Tony, and Seth Borenstein, "Fda's Approval Policy Pits Speed Against Safety," *The Philadelphia Inquirer*, December 23, 2004.

Schneider, Eric C., Alan M. Zaslavsky, and Arnold M. Epstein. "Racial Disparities in the Quality of Care for Enrollees in Medicare Managed Care." *Journal of American Medical Association* 287 (March 13, 2002): 1288–94.

Shute, Nancy, "That Old-Time Medicine," *U.S. News & World Report*, April 22, 2002.

Soumerai, Stephen, et al. "Adverse Outcomes of Underuse of Beta Blockers in Elderly Survivors of Acute Myocardial Infarction." *Journal of American Medical Association* 277 (1997): 115–21.

Spiegel, D., et al. "Effect Of Psychosocial Treatment on Survival of Patients with Metastatic Breast Cancer." *Lancet* 2 (October 14, 1989): 888–91.

Steve Findlay. *Prescription Drugs and Mass Media Advertising, 2000*. Washington, D.C.: National Institute for Health Care Management Foundation, November 21, 2001.

Stires, David, "Health Insurance: The Coming Crash in Health Care," *Fortune*, October 2, 2002.

U.S. Department of Health and Human Services. *Healthy People 2010: Understanding and Improving Health*. 2nd ed. vol. 2. Washington, D.C.: GPO, 2000.

U.S. Supreme Court Reports. *Kentucky Association of Health Plans, Inc., et al. v. Miller, Commissioner, Kentucky Department of Insurance*, 00–1471. Washington, D.C.: April 2, 2003.

U.S. Bureau of the Census. Current Population Reports. *Income, Poverty, and Health Insurance Coverage in the United States: 2003*. Washington, D.C.: August, 2004.

United Nations. *Report of the Second World Assembly on Aging*. ISBN 92-1-130221-8. New York: April 8–12, 2002.

Wootton, J.C., and A. Sparber, "Surveys of Complementary and Alternative Medicine: Part I. General Trends and Demographic Groups." *Journal of Alternative and Complementary Medicine* 7 (April 2001): 195–208.

Index

Activist Cancer Patient, The (Zakarian), 152
advance health care directive, 141–42, 148
advocates for patients/consumers, 32–33, 79, 106–7, 147–48, 150
alternative medicine. *See also* health information
 and commercialization, 12
 and conventional medicine, 22, 34–35, 78–79
 and elitism, medical, 13, 14–15, 18–19
 and emergency medical kits, 146
 and insurance industry, 138
 organizations, 184–88
 professional associations, 184–88
 and profits, 13, 15
 and records/reports, 78–79
 and regulation, 12, 13, 15
 and self-care, 98
 and standards, 12
 and time frame for healing, 31, 77
 and treatments, 124–25
alternative providers, 47–48, 66–67, 69, 77–78, 105–6
American Board of Medical Specialties, 49
American Medical Association, 17–18

appointments, medical
 and advocates, 79
 and assertive approach of patients/consumers, 74–75, 79–82
 check list, 69
 and communication with providers, 75–79
 and fees for services, 78
 and medical billing services, 73–74
 and medical jargon, 73–74
 and monitoring/mapping progress, 122
 and patient syndrome, 63–64
 and powerlessness issues, 72, 74
 and records/reports, 78–79
 and replacement of providers, 77–78
 scheduling, 78
assertiveness issues, 8, 35, 71–72, 74–75, 79–82, 81–82
Attention-Deficit/Hyperactivity Disorder (ADHD), 13

billing services, medical, 73–74

capitalism, and health care, 11–12
commercialization issues, 12
communication issues, 30, 75–79, 101–2
confidentiality issues, 16, 114, 131
Consumer Information Center, 114

conventional medicine
   and alternative medicine, 22, 34–35, 78–79
   and conventional medicine industry, 10, 14, 16, 46, 130, 156
   and elitism, medical, 13, 14–15, 18–19
   and malpractice claims, medical, 19–21, 31–32, 159
   organizations, 183–84
   and pharmaceutical industry, 14–15
   professional associations, 183–84
   and profits, 13, 14–15, 158
   and providers, health care, 10, 156
   and records/reports, 78–79
   and regulations, 10, 156
   and rights, health care, 129
   and self-care, 94
   and specialists, medical, 21–22
   and time frame for healing, 31, 77
costs of services, 58–59, 78
customer service, and providers, 50

diseases/illnesses, 29, 30, 83–84, 130. *See also* health information

economic issues, 14, 58–59, 78. *See also* profitability issues
education, health care. *See* information, health
elitism, medical, 13, 14–15, 18–19
emergencies, medical
   and active role of patients/consumers, 145, 153–54
   and advance health care directive, 141–42, 148
   and advocates, 147–48
   check list, 154
   and contact numbers, 146
   and hospitals, 149–51
   and household accidents, 146
   and information, health care, 149
   medical kits, 146
   and provider relationships, 147
   and rights, health care, 149
environmental issues, 14, 96–97
exercise issues, 94, 96

family nurse practitioners (FNP or NP), 102–3, 106–7
Federal Privacy Act of 1974, 114
Federal Trade Commission (FTC), 88
fees for services, 58–59, 78
Food and Drug Administration, 15, 27, 52, 91
Freedom of Information Act of 1966, 114

government, federal
   Department of Health and Human Services, 52, 91
   Drug Enforcement Agency, 51
   Federal Privacy Act of 1974, 114
   Federal Trade Commission (FTC), 88
   Food and Drug Administration, 15, 27, 52, 91
   Freedom of Information Act of 1966, 114
   Health and Human Services' Division of Quality Assurances, 50
   Health Insurance Portability and Accountability Act of 1996, 137
   Joint Commission on Accreditation of Healthcare Organizations (JCAHO), 52, 131–32, 151, 153
   National Institutes of Health (NIH), 15, 92
   resources, 90, 91–92, 167–80
   Your Right to Federal Records (Consumer Information Center), 114

Halkin, Katherine, *New Way to Take Charge of Your Medical Treatment*, 152–53

Index

Hardt, Barbara, *New Way to Take Charge of Your Medical Treatment,* 152–53
healers. *See* providers, health care
healing process, 29, 31, 77, 119–22
health care
   about, 156–57
   and active role of patients/consumers, 157, 159, 162, 163
   and advance health care directive, 141–42, 148
   and attitudes of patients/consumers, 95–96, 156, 159, 162
   and capitalism, 11–12
   and claims/frauds, 20–21, 31–32, 159
   and commercialization, 12
   complexities of, 157
   and confidentiality issues, 16, 114, 131
   and emergencies, medical, 149
   environment of, 9–10, 11, 23–24
   and errors, medical, 26–27
   inequities in, 13
   information about, 149
   and insurance health benefits, 10–11
   organizations, 52–53
   politicization of, 22–23
   and power/powerlessness issues, 34–35, 72, 74
   and profits, 13, 19, 151, 158
   and rights, 129
   and self-care, 94
   as service industry, 10
health consciousness, 25–26
health information
   and active role of patients/consumers, 157–58
   diseases/illnesses research, 30, 83–84
   government resources, 90, 91–92, 167–80
   and hospitals's resources for patients/consumers, 152
   Internet resources, 85–89, 110, 133, 149
   libraries and bookstores, 90
   medical information services, 89–90, 181–82
   and networks for patients/consumers, 110
   resources, 84–85
Health Insurance Portability and Accountability Act of 1996, 137
health maintenance organization (HMO), 16, 46, 130
hormonal replacement therapy (HRT), 13
hospitals
   and active role of patients/consumers, 150–51
   check lists, 151–52
   and conventional medicine industry, 10, 14, 16, 46, 130, 156
   and emergencies, medical, 149–51
   and hospitalists, 150
   and information resources for patients/consumers, 152
   and medical support staff, 150, 151
   and patient safety officers, 151
   and profitability issues, 151
   and providers, health care, 10, 156
   and regulations, 10
   and safety standards, 131–32, 151
   Take This Book to the Hospital with You (Inlander), 152

illnesses, 13, 29, 30, 83–84, 130. *See also* health information
information, health. *See* health information
   and patients/consumers, 160
Inlander, Charles, *Take This Book to the Hospital with You,* 152
Institute of Medicine, 13, 27
insurance industry
   and alternative medicine, 138
   and benefits, health care, 10–11
   and confidentiality issues, 16
   Health Insurance Portability

and Accountability Act
of 1996, 137
and managed care, 16, 17,
18–19
and medical decision, 17
National Association
of Insurance
Commissioners, 133
and profits, 16–17
and rights, health care, 132,
135–38, 139
vs. providers, 15–16
Internet resources, 85–89, 110,
133, 149

jargon, medical, 73–74
Joint Commission on
Accreditation of Healthcare
Organizations (JCAHO), 52,
131–32, 151, 153

legal issues. *See also* government,
federal; insurance industry;
regulations; rights, health
care
and claims/frauds, 20–21,
31–32, 159
and legislation of health care
rights, 130
and mandatory benefit laws,
132–33
medical malpractice claims,
19–21, 31–32, 159
lifestyle habits, 30, 93–94, 95–96

Making Them Pay (Orin), 143
malpractice claims, medical,
19–21, 31–32, 159
managed care industry, 16, 17,
18–19, 131
mapping progress of healing, 31,
119–22
Maugham, W. Somerset, 8
Mead, Margaret, 35
Medicaid, 137
medical appointments. *See*
appointments, medical
Medical Information Board (MIB),
116

Medical Records: Getting Yours
(Public Citizen Health
Research Group), 114
Medicare, 18, 137
monitoring/mapping progress of
healing, 31, 119–22

Nader, Ralph, 12
National Academy of Sciences, 26
National Association of Insurance
Commissioners, 133
National Institutes of Health
(NIH), 15, 92
National Practitioner's Data Bank
(NPDB), 50–51
networks of patients/consumers,
30, 109–12
*New Way to Take Charge of Your
Medical Treatment* (Hardt
and Halkin), 152–53

organizations. *See also specific
organizations*
and alternative medicine,
184–88
conventional medicine, 183–84
government resources, 90,
91–92, 167–80
and rights, health care, 143–44,
181–82
Orin, Rhonda, *Making Them Pay*, 143

patients/consumers. *See also*
appointments, medical
active role of, 25–27, 29–31,
159–60
assertive approach of, 8, 35,
71–72, 74–75, 79–82
attitudes of, 95–96, 156, 159,
162
as consumers, 27–29, 63–64,
80–81
and education, health, 160
and errors, medical, 26–27, 27
and health consciousness,
25–26
and patient syndrome, 63–64
and power/powerlessness
issues, 34–35, 72, 74

Index

quiz, 37–44
and racial issues, 13
and records/reports, 30, 117
and relationships with
  providers, 147
and time frame for healing,
  31, 77
and victims, health care, 31–32,
  37–44
and women's issues, 13
pharmaceutical industry, 14–15
physician assistants (PA), 103, 107
power/powerlessness issues, 34–35,
  72, 74
Preferred Provider networks (PPO),
  46
privacy issues, 16, 114, 131
professional associations, 183–88
profitability issues
  and alternative medicine, 13,
    15
  and conventional medicine,
    13, 14–15, 158
  and healers, 17
  and health care, 13, 19, 151,
    158
  and hospitals, 151
  and insurance industry, 16–17
  and providers, health care,
    17–18, 158
  and salaries of providers, 17–18
providers, health care
  and active role of patients/
    consumers, 161–62
  and assertive approach of
    patients/consumers, 8,
    35, 71–72, 74–75, 79–82
  and capability issues, 57
  check list for choosing, 69
  choosing, 29–30, 45–48
  and claims/frauds, 20–21,
    31–32, 159
  and competency, 48–50
  and conservatism, 58
  consultations with, 53–54
  and conventional medicine
    industry, 10, 156
  and customer service, 50
  and disciplinary actions, 50–52

discussion topics for visits with,
  64–66
and drug/substance abuse
  issues, 50
expectations about, 59–60
and fees for services, 58–59
and hospitals, 10
intentions of, 55–57
and malpractice claims,
  medical, 19–21
and medical decisions, 17
and patient compliance, 29
and patient syndrome, 63–64
preparation for visits with,
  63–64, 66–69
and profits, 17–18, 158
and relationships with
  patients/consumers, 147
replacement of, 77–78
and second opinions, 68
selecting, 54–55, 60–61
sensitivity of, 73
types of, 46–47
Public Citizen Health Research
  Group, 114

racial issues, 13
records/reports, 30, 78–79, 113–17
regulations. See also legal issues
  and alternative medicine, 12,
    13, 15
  and conventional medicine
    industry, 10, 156
  and hospitals, 10
  and medical decisions, 17
research, health care. See
  information, health
rights, health care
  and active role of patients/
    consumers, 31, 133–35
  and advance health care
    directive, 141–42, 148
  check lists, 133–35, 144
  and claims, 138–40, 159
  and confidentiality issues, 16,
    114, 131
  and consumer advocacy
    groups, 143–44, 181–82
  and conventional medicine, 129

and drug addiction, 130
and emergencies, medical, 149
and environment of health care, 24
information on, 142–43
and insurance industry, 132, 135–38, 139
Internet resources, 133
legislation of, 130
and mandatory benefit laws, 132
and mental illness, 130
organizations, 143–44, 181–82
and providers, health care, 46, 138–39
and safety standards, 131–32, 151
and self-determination, 130
and taxes, 140–41

safety standards, 131–32, 151
self-care
and active role of patients/consumers, 30, 93, 98–99
and alternative medicine, 98
and attitudes of patients/consumers, 95–96
check list, 99
and conventional medicine, 94
and environmental issues, 96–97
and exercise, 94, 96
and health care, 94
and lifestyle habits, 30, 93–94, 95–96
and medicines, 97–98
and records/reports, 122
and self-determination, 130
and stress management, 95
and treatments, 95
service industry, and health care, 10
standards issues, 12, 131–32
stress management, 95
support issues
advocates for patients/consumers, 32–33, 79, 106–7, 147–48, 150
medical support staff, 101–5, 106–7, 150, 151

and social support, 109–10, 111–12
syndrome, patient, 63–64

Take This Book to the Hospital with You (Inlander), 152
technology, and environmental issues, 14
treatments
and active role of patients/consumers, 30, 76–79
and alternative medicine, 124–25
and attitudes of patients/consumers, 125–26
and benefits of healing process, 121–22
New Way to Take Charge of Your Medical Treatment (Hardt and Halkin), 152–53
and observations during healing process, 120–21, 122
and patience of patients/consumers, 123–27
and self-care, 95

U.S. Department of Health and Human Services, 52, 91
U.S. Drug Enforcement Agency, 51
U.S. Federal Trade Commission (FTC), 88
U.S. Food and Drug Administration, 15, 27, 52, 91
U.S. Health and Human Services' Division of Quality Assurances, 50

women's issues, 13

Your Right to Federal Records (Consumer Information Center), 114

Zakarian, Beverly, *The Activist Cancer Patient,* 152